EYE MOVEMENTS, VISION AND BEHAVIOR

A HIERARCHICAL VISUAL INFORMATION PROCESSING MODEL

KENNETH R. GAARDER

Department of Psychiatry
University of Texas Health Science Center at San Antonio

and

Clinical Psychophysiology Service
Audie L. Murphy Memorial Veterans Administration Hospital
San Antonio, Texas

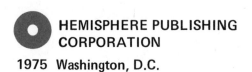 HEMISPHERE PUBLISHING
CORPORATION
1975 Washington, D.C.

A HALSTED PRESS BOOK

JOHN WILEY & SONS
New York   London   Sydney   Toronto

Hemisphere Publishing Corporation
1025 Vermont Avenue, N.W., Washington, D.C. 20005

Distributed solely by Halsted Press, a Division of John Wiley & Sons, Inc., New York.

Library of Congress Cataloging in Publication Data:

Gaarder, Kenneth R
    Eye movements, vision, and behavior,

    1. Eye—Movements. 2. Vision. 3. Information
theory in biology. I. Title. [DNLM: 1. Behavior.
2. Eye movements. 3. Visual perception. WW103 Gllle]
QP477.5.G3   612'.846   74-14710
ISBN 0-470-28895-7
Printed in the United States of America

For Marie, Jason, and Galen

CONTENTS

FOREWORD

We live in an era of evolutionary dynamics and of experimental-quantitative method. This means that in every work of psychological research we must ask whether the perspective is broad and the methodology sophisticated. To grasp the psychology of the perceptual act—as in reading a book—we must understand how the eyes, the brain, and the muscles actually work; how the living system as a whole is expressed in the dynamic of the quantum or "all-or-none" law; and how the resulting "step functions," in hierarchical order, bring to the organism the orderly and meaningful information that forms the basis for the difference between adaptation and adaptive failure. It turns out that information-theory has edged its way into a dominant position in the field of perception research.

These are some of the reasons why Dr. Gaarder's book, informed and profoundly oriented to these issues, can be intensely exciting to a psychologist. Whether he is anchored in a classic Helmholtzian viewpoint or guided by allegiance to the modern concepts of step-function and quanta, or drawn into the whirling vortex of information-theory he will come to view retina, eye muscle, and brain as elements of a system of adaptive sequences.

But there is one more modern concept which pushes its way to the center of the stage. From the engineer's servomechanism to Claude Bernard's *milieu intérieur* one great actor in the modern drama has made its way forward to demand a central place: and this is the conception of *feedback*. To be sure, the feedback concept is to be found back there in Helmholtz and in

Sherrington. But with Cannon and with homeostasis it has become a *leitmotif*, a focus of psychophysiology and a recurrent center of emphasis in modern experimental research. The synthesis of all these ideas is one of the things which make Dr. Gaarder's book both important and exciting.

Gardner Murphy

George Washington University

PREFACE

The purpose of this book is to describe explicitly and completely the model of visual information processing which emerges from a thorough consideration of the role of eye movements in perception. Prior analyses have not carried the examination of the simple physical facts (as opposed to the interpretable experimental data) to the stark and revealing conclusion possible. Science is a confusing mixture of complexity and simplicity and one of the scientist's jobs is to seek simplicity when it is appropriate. Doing so does not reduce the overall complexity of the field, but does increase the validity of the immediate mapping of reality by models.

Herein, we take a few experimental facts, combined with the geometrical and physical facts of what happens when the eye moves, and show how a solid and lucid picture of visual information processing emerges. As soon as one gives appropriate weight to the simple facts, the conclusions become apparent.

Visual information processing is shown to be a discontinuous, hierarchically organized process structured by jumping eye movements. Further speculative conclusions about information processing in general are appended in Chaps. 7 and 8 to demonstrate the wider impact of the model. These, however, are apart from, and beyond, the main model of the visual information processing and do not affect its validity.

The book is intended both as a monograph in the field of eye movements and vision, and as a textbook suitable for supplemental assigments in courses on physiological psychology, vision, and biological information processing. The style, as well as the content, deliberately seeks simplicity and clarity. Effort has been made to lay a foundation for and define all the unfamiliar ideas introduced. The book is organized to build progressively from one chapter to the next, with each chapter having its major focus upon the issue named in the chapter title. Those who wish to know the central theme of the book before considering how conclusions were reached can begin with Chap. 6 and then return to the earlier chapters, while those desiring a concise statement of the arguments can begin with Chap. 9. People already familiar with a particular area may be able to comprehend the gist of a chapter by skimming, but most readers will find it desirable to proceed through the book following the sequential order of the chapters.

Kenneth R. Gaarder

November 1974

ACKNOWLEDGMENTS

Many people have contributed to the work reported in this book. In the early stages, the late Cyrus P. Barnum, Jr., Alfred Stanton, Harold Levitan, Julius Korien, the late Gordon Walls, and Gregory Bateson all influenced and encouraged me. The first experimental work was done at the Langley Porter division of the University of California Medical Center in a program headed by Enoch Callaway and Jurgen Ruesch. Chester Trent, Tom Cornsweet, and Alex Sweet made crucial contributions to that work.

Dexter Bullard, Marvin Adland, and Donald L. Burnham at Chestnut Lodge in Rockville, Maryland, made it possible to continue vision work by providing from Ford Foundation funds that paradoxical necessity of our modern era—a grant to support my applying for a larger grant. For two years my work was then supported by Public Health Service grant MH06554-01. Chestnut Lodge also brought me into contact with David Rioch, who made it possible to work in the vision laboratory of John Armington, in an ideal scientific environment for several years. My colleagues, William Biersdorf, Robert Chapman, Allen Granda, John Krauskopf, and Richard Srebro gave generously of their time and help and I had the opportunity to work with members of the supporting staff and graduate students: Henry Bragdon, Joseph Fritz, Virgil Graf, Walter Kropfl, Abner Lall, Harold Lawson, Allison Lee, Marco Montemezzi, Edward Olechowski, and Joseph Scott, who was the subject in the audiovisual interaction experiment.

My period of work at the National Institute of Mental Health branch at St. Elizabeths Hospital was supported by Robert Cohen, whose administrative style I greatly admire, and Joel Elkes and Fritz Freyhan, who helped in every way possible. From Dr. Freyhan's successor, Gian-Carlo Salmoiraghi, I acquired most of my present knowledge of higher level Federal administrative procedures. My assistants, Richard Koresco and Arthur Alterman, were invaluable to the work reported, and Ruth Wise provided highly competent secretarial skills. The most valuable part of the time at St. Elizabeths was the opportunity to work with Louise Speck, Stephen Szara, Margaret Mercer, and Larry Frost in a seminar where we absorbed W. Ross Ashby's *Introduction to Cybernetics*. We worked hard together and what I gained has been integral to my thinking in this book. During that period I also worked closely with the technical departments at the National Institutes of Health in the design of equipment and in the use of their computers. Here James Bryan, Leo Leitner, Richard Newell, Norwood Simmons, and William Sheriff were helpful in various capacities. I also had the opportunity to work with Julian Silverman and his staff—Catherine King and Dolf and Louise Pfefferbaum. Figures which show the effects of eye movements resulted from collaboration between Martin Finch, medical artist, Lee Bragg of the photographic service, and me.

While working at the Veterans Administration Hospital in Washington, D.C., I worked at Walter Reed through the kindness of Thomas Frazier, who had succeeded John Armington.

Others involved have not been attached to these institutions. They include Isabelle Kendig, who has provided valuable criticism; John Kafka, who has been a good friend and intellectual provocateur; George Nesbitt and Gardner Murphy, who have read and commented on this manuscript; and Verdelia Scott, Sally Minshew, and Linda Huff, who typed the manuscripts.

The work on the manuscript was done while at the University of Texas Health Science Center at San Antonio and the Audie L. Murphy Memorial Veterans Administration Hospital with the cooperation of Robert Leon, Edward Krollar, and Augustin de la Peña. Opinions expressed in this book do not reflect the policies of these institutions.

Finally, a most important contribution has been the emotional support, encouragement, and patience of my wife, Marie, and our sons, Jason and Galen, who have been with me during the work.

1
FEEDBACK IN VISION

1.1. Introduction

The concept of feedback is a major focus around which modern biology has been reorganized. A central purpose of this book is to show specifically how feedback is crucial to the act of visual perception. This will be done by concretely demonstrating how the feedback caused by eye movements moving the image upon the retina is essential to the process by which visual information is taken into the central nervous system. The entire picture of this process will emerge in later chapters.

To show how feedback affects vision we will first describe feedback more thoroughly as a general process and as a biological process; this will be done in Chap. 1. The latter part of the chapter will then present logical and experimental evidence demonstrating the feedback provided by eye movements.

FEEDBACK AS A GENERAL ISSUE

1.2. Survival, Adaptation, and Homeostasis as Biological Axioms

Before considering feedback as an issue, it is well to consider why feedback is so important. Feedback is the mechanism mediating the adaptive process of homeostasis. Since the time of Darwin, man has experienced the impact of the idea that organisms are adaptive; they are designed to survive.

The pervasiveness of this theme in modern biological and cybernetic thinking is shown in hundreds of scientific titles referring to adaptation; the power of the argument that adaptation is biologically axiomatic has been eloquently demonstrated by Ashby (1963, p. 197) who shows that survival is the first task of adaptation and that the common heritage of all living organisms is their descent from those ancestors who survived.

Survival and adaptation are mediated by *homeostasis.* This elegant physiological concept was anticipated by the French physiologist, Claude Bernard, in the last century and elaborated by Walter Cannon during the first decade of this century. Homeostasis refers to the biological necessity of maintaining certain physiological variables within adaptive limits for the purpose of survival (Langley, 1965). There are hundreds of such variables that can be identified in an organism—body temperature is one example and the specific levels of many elements of the blood such as oxygen, salt, sugar, and protein are others.

Consideration of body temperature as an example can clarify the concept. We know that human survival is not possible when internal body temperature varies too many degrees from 98°F and that it is possible for the human organism to maintain this relatively constant body temperature despite wide swings of external temperature. Homeostasis is the organizing concept that acknowledges the relative constancy of the variable, the failure of survival with too great change of the variable, the adaptive function of maintaining the variable, and the need to explain the mechanism for maintaining the variable. The essential feature of a homeostatic mechanism is that some particular variable is kept from going above or below critical limits as a contribution to the equilibrium of the body as a whole. The overall picture of homeostasis within the organism is one of many forces being in a harmonious balance with one another.

This leads to a comparison between the concept of homeostasis and the concept of holism in which one attempts to consider a system as a whole rather than as a mere aggregate of its parts. Holistic psychologies—such as those offered by Cantril (1950), Dewey (1922), Lewin (1936), Mead (1938), and Schilder (1950, p. 151)—have presented strong arguments showing the inadequacy of piecemeal approaches, but have foundered upon their own failure to relate to specific physiological mechanism. Homeostasis offers a way of reconciling the comprehensiveness of holistic viewpoints with the physiological specificity of piecemeal approaches.

Psychology is now undergoing reorganization around the recognition of the need to consider the organism as a whole and in relation to its environment while at the same time specifying physiological mechanisms. The concepts of adaptation and homeostasis are not only relevant physiologically, but are acknowledged as psychological necessities as well in the thinking of such leaders as Murphy (1966); the general systems theorist von Bertalanffy (1967); and Sokolov (1963). Murphy, as an American eclectic and pragmatist, must account for any such seminal ideas; while for Sokolov, in the Russian tradition, it is taken as the psychologist's main task to explain how man adapts to his environment, and from Pavlov, to explain the detailed mechanism as a process.

1.3. Feedback as the Mediator of Homeostasis

Although concepts of feedback, as embodied in such mechanisms as Watt's steam engine governor, are at least as old as concepts of adaptation and homeostasis (Mayr, 1970), only recently has it become clear that the particular mechanism mediating adaptive homeostasis is feedback. Thus, these general concepts—adaptation and homeostasis—reflecting the organism's relationship to its environment and the relationship between particular attributes of the organism, must be explained by this other more specific concept (Langley, 1965). I shall not demonstrate this fact here, but will instead proceed into a more thorough discussion of feedback.

1.4. The Taxonomy of Feedback

Feedback can be categorized in several ways. The simplest is to consider cybernetics as the science that studies feedback and its principles generally and to divide feedback systems into those in living systems and those in nonliving systems. The principles of feedback in nonliving systems have been thoroughly and rigorously studied. Wiener (1948) and others attribute the elaboration of the principles of the nonliving feedback system to electrical engineers who developed the vacuum tube for radio use during the 1930s and to the result of scientific effort in World War II for such purposes as the radar controlled antiaircraft gun control system. Although specific living feedback systems had been studied earlier, under the inspiration of Wiener it began to become clear that the understanding of living system feedback placed a rich and powerful conceptual tool in the hands of biological scientists. Many of the principles of feedback in nonliving systems apply to living systems as well, but others do not. In addition, the understanding of biological feedback has not yet been reduced to coherent known and generally accepted principles. Current tasks of cybernetics are to determine general principles which apply to all feedback systems and to elaborate special principles for living systems.

Here will follow a brief summary of those principles that have been well established; then feedback in the visual system can be studied.

1.5. The Central Concept of Feedback

The basic idea of feedback is demonstrated by the steam engine governor, whose purpose is to maintain the speed of the engine constant (Fig. 1.1). In its familiar form, the flywheel of the engine transmits power (A) to an axle (B), around which spin heavy weights (C). The faster the engine goes, the further out centrifugal force carries the weights. The slower the engine goes the more gravity carries the weights downward and close to the axle. The motion of the weights is transmitted by levers (D) to control the flow of steam (E) to the engine (F). If the engine speeds up, the mechanism causes the flow of steam to be cut back, thereby in turn slowing the engine; on the other hand, if the engine slows down, the flow of steam is increased, thereby causing the engine to go faster. Thus, the speed of the engine is maintained relatively constant by these adjustments. While it is straightforward to understand that the steam pressure to the engine controls the speed of the engine (Fig. 1.2), by using a governor the more complex situation of feedback has been created; feedback derived from the speed of the engine in turn controls the steam pressure going to the engine (Fig. 1.3). Although the mechanics and the concept of feedback, as exemplified by a governor, are both simple, it is important to realize that the concept is elusive.

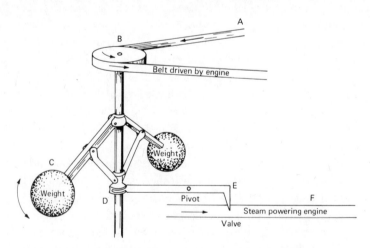

Fig. 1.1. Steam engine governor with negative feedback.
Higher Speed (+) ⟶ Lower Steam Pressure (−)
Lower Speed (−) ⟶ Higher Steam Pressure (+)

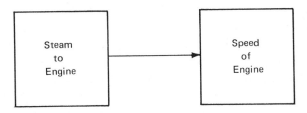

Fig. 1.2. Block diagram of control without feedback.

1.6. Characteristics of Feedback Systems

It is beyond the scope of this book to describe here in detail the general principles of feedback; these principles have been dealt with elsewhere (Jones, 1973; Navweps OP3000, 1963; Ritow, 1963). Instead of dealing with principles, which would involve mathematical descriptions of feedback, I shall describe some characteristics of feedback systems and refer the interested reader to other sources.

Feedback Systems Can Be Described by Block Diagrams. By using boxes to represent physical entities and arrows to represent channels capable of transmitting energy and information, a new "language" has been developed which communicates essential features of feedback systems. (See Figs. 1.2, 1.3, 1.7, & 1.8.) The use of block diagrams is carried still further by electronic engineers and computer programmers, but the formal properties of the language thereby created has not yet been studied extensively.

Feedback Systems Are Closed Loop Systems. One feature of the block diagram of a feedback system is that the boxes and the arrows eventually form a closed circle and "close the loop." This is necessary but not sufficient to define a feedback in a block diagram, since all closed loops are not feedback.

Negative Feedbacks Tend to Promote Stability. The mathematical description of a feedback as positive or negative is one of its most crucial

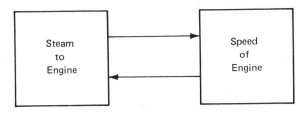

Fig. 1.3. Block diagram of feedback control.

determinants. Referring to Fig. 1.1, notice that the governor stabilizes the engine's speed because it always causes an effect in the opposite (negative) direction from that of the changes in the engine's speed—if the engine speeds up (increase), the governor cuts off steam (decrease), slowing the engine. It is the fact that the feeedback is in the opposite (negative) direction from the original effect that causes it to stabilize the situation. Stability is not an inevitable result of negative feedback, because other factors may still make the system unstable.

Most living system feedbacks thus far analyzed are negative feedback systems tending toward stability and it should be kept in mind that these are the systems referred to as homeostatic.

Positive Feedbacks Promote Instability. A situation where positive feedback operates causes instability of the system. We can use a steam engine governor with the lever linkages reversed (Fig. 1.4) as an example. Now a *higher* speed of the engine causes *higher* steam pressure (positive feedback), which drives the engine still faster, while a *lower* speed of the engine causes *lower* steam pressure, and the engine slows still further. This positive feedback is an inherently unstable linkage that always moves in a particular direction once triggered. Many living system feedbacks are positive.These have been described in psychological systems by Wender (1968) as deviation-amplifying feedback, by Ashby (1963, p. 81) with an apparent exception to the instability of positive feedback, and by Iberall and McCulloch (1968)

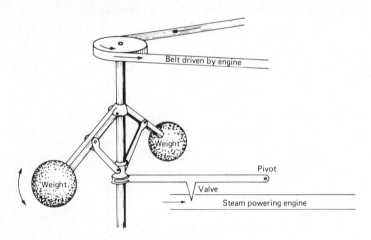

Fig. 1.4.   Steam engine governor with positive feedback.
Higher Speed (+) ⟶ Higher Steam Pressure (+)
Lower Speed (−) ⟶ Lower Steam Pressure (−)

where instability is conceptualized as *homeokinesis,* drawing attention to the fact that the stability of homeostasis as a characteristic of living systems should not blind us to the frequent occurrence of instability as an adaptive process. Thus, a primary function of positive feedback is to cause an organism to react adaptively to a stimulus by drastically changing in some crucial respect. (See Sec. 1.11.)

Feedback Systems Have Steady State and Dynamic Descriptions. The static description of a feedback system merely tells what elements are connected and how they are connected. For this a block diagram may suffice. The dynamic description tells what the system does under specific conditions. This involves mathematical descriptions which are often visualized graphically (Ritow, 1963).

Feedback Systems Are Affected by Time Delays. An immediately apparent problem is analyzing any feedback system is the consideration of the time it takes for transmission of information. For example, when a steam engine slows down, it takes time to overcome inertia before the weights fall which open the steam valve wider, and it takes still more time for the increased steam pressure to affect the engine. This means that the response of the governor to increase the steam pressure is always a few moments late. Among other things, this can lead to the engine speeding up and slowing down, since a given correction is never correct for that moment but always for a moment before. This is visualized graphically in Fig. 1.5 where one sinusoidal curve represents steam pressure and the other represents engine speed. The discrepancy between the two curves is technically known as a phase lag, i.e., there is a time lag between the phases of the two sinusoidal waves representing the changes of speed and steam pressure. The mathematical laws needed to understand and control the problems thus created have been worked out and are well known to engineers (Ritow, 1963). In living systems there are similar time delays analogous to phase lags. For example, when a light flashes on the retina of the eye, there are variable time delays before the message reaches the cortex of the brain because of the time it takes for nerve signals to pass down a nerve and the additional time it takes the signal to go from one nerve cell to the next at the junction between nerves.

Feedback Systems Have Particular Stability Characteristics. Engineers are able to take precise measurements of the major variables of a feedback system and determine the stability of the system under various circumstances. Among the more important variables to be considered in determining stablity are gain, phase lag, and positivity versus negativity of feedback. Gain is the relationship of the feedback signal amplitude to the original signal amplitude.

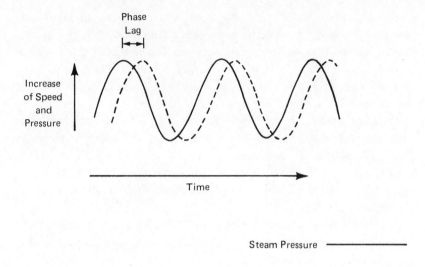

Fig. 1.5. Phase lag.

An engineer might analyze a steam engine governor and tell that if it is set for a speed of 300 revolutions per minute it would have the optimal stability of engine speed, whereas if the governor were set for a speed of 150 revolutions per minute there would be bothersome slowing and speeding up. He might also tell what loads on the engine would disturb its stability at different speeds by changing phase relationships. Some of the possible types of stability are pictured in self-explanatory terms in Fig. 1.6.

Feedback Systems Are Limited by Their Channel Capacities. In the simple and idealized systems thus far considered there are no problems of the feedback linkages being inadequate to convey required information between components. In complex real systems and especially in parsimonious biological systems, however, the feedback linkage, which is technically an information channel, has a limit in its capacity to carry information. Ashby's Law of Requisite Variety (1963, p. 206) shows how the degree of control achievable by a feedback system is determined by the channel capacity of the feedback linkage and how stabilized feedback control will not be achieved if the variety (a technical term for information quantity) of the disturbances effectively causing unique alterations of the system is greater than the variety of the stabilizing feedback information channel (Conant, 1969).

Feedback Systems Have Linear or Nonlinear Properties. Here is usually one of the major distinctions between living and nonliving feedback systems.

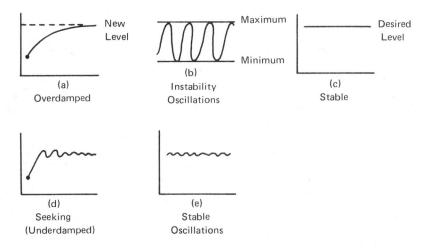

Fig. 1.6. Schematic illustrations of various possible types of stability characteristics.

In mathematics, a linear relation between two functions means that the plot of the functions on a graph is a straight line. Linear relationships are relatively simpler and are generalizable from case to case. Many nonliving feedback systems are linear and follow rigorous general laws which, though complex, are thoroughly understood by engineers.

On the other hand, living feedback systems tend to be nonlinear. This means that the relationship between two functions cannot be expressed as a straight line, but must be some form of curved line—such as a ∪ or ∩ or an S-shaped line, etc. Nonlinear relationships can not be generalized across groups; they are relatively more complex, and often cannot be deciphered and reduced to mathematical form in a meaningful way.

The importance of this is that while nonliving feedback systems are usually well understood and can be analyzed by the application of general principles, each type of living feedback system must usually be considered a case unto itself, requiring its own special, often arduous analysis. There is not yet a general systems theory of feedback to be meaningfully applied to living feedback systems.

1.7. Special Issues Concerning Living Feedback Systems

Ashby (1963, p 4) has proposed that analogy is one of the most powerful means of reasoning, and it is universally acknowledged that biological science is heavily dependent upon a process in which there is repeated comparison between the particular system studied, the abstract scientific model of the system, and the larger "pool" or set of models taken from all similar systems—living and nonliving. Because we reason by analogy, we will draw upon concepts from a number of fields in our modeling. It is here that we encounter both the concrete nonliving feedback systems and the abstract laws explaining these systems. The laws of presently existing nonliving feedback systems are well worked out and thoroughly studied; while the laws of living feedback systems are not nearly so well understood. At the same time, it must be recognized that the concept of feedback mechanisms in living systems may be one of the richest organizers of advancing knowledge.

Another problem met here is the problem of hierarchy—to be dealt with in more detail in Chap. 5. At the lowest hierarchical level are the simplest elements—receptor, nerve, and muscle cells; and the models are the most concrete. To model at higher hierarchical levels, larger, more abstract and less knowable entities must be dealt with—the retina, the optic nerve, brain structures, etc.—and the models are more abstract and yet at the same time more relevant to the immediate concerns of man. Von Foerster (1971 p. 1) has posed this as the dilemma encountered after reduction in his Theorem Number Two: "The hard sciences are successful because they deal with the soft problems; the soft sciences are struggling because they deal with the hard problems." Scientific explanation can also be thought of as being satisfactory in varying degrees, becoming more and more immediately satisfactory as it becomes more and more specific.

1.8. Study of Living Feedback Systems

Feedback, as the mediating mechanism of homeostasis (which in turn assures adaptation and survival), is a central concept of modern biology. Its place therein is dealt with by Chase (1965); Clark (1963); Jones (1973); Powers (1973); Powers, Clark, and McFarland (1960); Stark (1968); Thomas (1970); von Bertalanffy (1968); Wender (1968); and Wiener (1948) among others. Feedback has been shown to operate in most biological mechanisms at all levels of abstraction. Thus, it is used as an explanation of mechanisms for establishing the balance between various chemical components of the body in metabolic reactions (Reiner, 1968); for regulating muscle reflex arcs (Chase, 1965; Granit, 1970); and for understanding gross behavior (Clark, 1963; Ruesch & Bateson, 1951; Sokolov, 1963; Wender, 1968).

1.9. Strategies for Studying Living
   System Feedback

A few years ago, before the concept of feedback had become well established, a major question in the analysis of a biological system was whether or not feedback was present. This is the sort of question that can often be answered rigorously, and although today the presence of feedback would too often be taken for granted without evidence, the pursuit of a sound answer is still justified. An analogous issue in the history of science was the question asked near the end of the last century of whether a microorganism was responsible for a particular disease. This question was answered by Koch's postulates: in order to consider a microorganism the cause of a disease it must be present in every case of the disease; it must be capable of cultivation in pure culture; it must, when inoculated in pure culture, produce the disease in susceptible animals; and it must be recoverable from the animal and again grown in pure culture.

A similar set of criteria can be established for demonstrating that feedback operates between two parts of a system. However, it remains for a logical consensus to be developed as to reasonable criteria. Instead, it must presently be accepted that the presence of a feedback can be demonstrated with greater and lesser degrees of certainty and with greater and lesser degrees of acceptability to other scientists.

Some criteria for demonstrating a feedback are: (a) whether tangible and operable connections exists in both directions between the two parts in question (see Secs. 1.12, 1.13, 1.15); (b) whether stimulation of one part causes a reaction in that part which can only be explained by reference to the connections between it and the other part; (c) whether stimulation of a part causes a reaction in an effector channel returning to that part (see Sec. 1.13); (d) whether stimulation of a part elicits a different reaction depending upon the state of the other part (see Sec. 1.20); (e) whether interrupting a channel between the two parts causes a part to react differently upon stimulation (consider stabilized retinal image experiments, Alpern, 1972).

The apparently simple analysis of these apparently straightforward questions is complicated by the fact that a consensually validated model of the feedback process has not yet been clarified scientifically; also, experimental evidence is often explainable by alternate hypotheses (Worden, 1966).

Once feedback between two parts is demonstrated, the next task is to demonstrate the operating characteristics of the feedback. This involves a number of steps, including identification of the elements in the feedback circuit, e.g., an initial experimental model to demonstrate a connection may designate two parts known to be connected and show the effect of one upon the other, but not specify the chain of connections. It then becomes a later task to do this. Further steps include testing the system under various conditions and determining: (a) stability and instability of the system;

(*b*) positivity versus negativity of the feedback; (*c*) the characteristics of the parts of the system: channel capacity, gain, response curves, etc; (*d*) the responses of the system as a whole: time lags, linear versus nonlinear responses, etc. Some of these issues will become clearer by considering feedback in the visual system.

FEEDBACK IN THE VISUAL SYSTEM

1.10.   The Adaptive Function of Vision

The adaptive function of vision is so obvious that it might easily be overlooked or reduced to triviality or a useless truism. The reader need only remind himself of the plight of the suddenly blind to recognize that the loss of vision in an organism adapted to its environment through vision can be catastrophic, even fatal. Generally, vision in a visually adapted organism is essential to such functions as locomotion, guiding movements of the limbs and head, self-protection, and interpreting the environment.

In man, there are in addition special functions, particularly reading, that enrich and complicate his adaptations. Thus, the entire life career of the child with an untreated reading disability may be impoverished. Finally, I shall show how many of the homeostatic mechanisms (referred to in the material that follows) are adaptive because they facilitate vision.

1.11.   Homeostasis in Vision

Earlier in this chapter you saw how adaptive functions are often mediated by homeostasis. Now, I will examine some of the ways in which homeostasis operates in the visual system. Although the concept of homeostasis in the visual system is nearly universally accepted, it is often only acknowledged implicitly and many discussions of clearly homeostatic mechanisms will not mention the term and will only use the concept implicitly.

One of the major homeostatic functions of vision is to maintain perceptual defenses: mechanisms whereby we do not perceive what we find threatening. Perceptual defenses have been studied by a number of investigators, including Luborsky, Rick, Phoenix, and Fisher (1968) and Singer, Greenberg, and Antrobus, (1971), and have been reviewed by Solley and Murphy (1960). The idea of perceptual defense can be grasped in the example of someone who does not wish to acknowledge violence in the world. His internal stability and equanimity are threatened when he is exposed to violence, and he often will be successful in so structuring his world that he does not have to deal with violence. Under a number of environmental conditions in which evidence of violence is present, such a person will selectively exclude the evidence. This might take a number of specific forms: reading a newspaper and only "seeing" headlines of nonviolent events; failing to notice when children fight; misreading tachistoscopically presented pictures of violence as nonviolent; etc. Although there are undoubtedly many physiological mechanisms involved in perceptual defenses and the mechanisms have not been worked out, the concept is well established through experimentation using behavioral evidence.

Another related homeostatic function of vision is maintaining a particular preferred level of physiological arousal. Arousal is a concept designating the degree of alertness or activation or "awakeness" of an organism. The degree of arousal is mediated in the brain by the reticular activating system. Soviet psychologists have extensively demonstrated the homeostasis of arousal level and Sokolov (1963) covered the subject well. A clear example is the case of habituation of responses, in which a particular stimulus will cause a marked reaction with heightened arousal the first few times applied, but with the reaction rapidly diminishing with succesive applications of the stimulus. This is adaptive and homeostatic in the following way: One of the major needs of all animal organisms is to escape danger, so that when a new stimulus appears in the animal's environment it is essential that it be analyzed immediately to determine if it represents danger. Thus, initially, a maximal response is desirable (homeokinesis). However, once the stimulus has been analyzed it is often determined that it does not mean danger and can safely be ignored. Now it is adaptive for the organism not to respond. Thus, to the first few stimuli, there is a large reaction with arousal, which through habituation is successively attenuated with return of the arousal level to the prestimulus level. Heightened arousal upon stimulation with subsequent habitation is characteristic of many visual system reaction, such as reactions to light-on or light-off stimuli, or to moving patterns. In another example of homeostasis of arousal, Palmer (1966, 1970) has shown how nearsightedness has the adaptive function of lowering chronic arousal level by always presenting a slightly defocused image for processing. Boernstein (1967) has also dealt with the homeostatic function of arousal, but in relation to dark adaptation.

Specific mechanisms where homeostasis has been demonstrated in the visual system include the ability to adjust to drastic changes of light level (light and dark adaptation); the ability to retain central foveal vision on a moving object (tracking); the ability to keep both eyes on a near object (convergence); the ability to keep the eyes on a stationary target (fixation); the ability to change the focal length of the lens of the eyes (accommodation); the ability to change the diameter of the pupil under changing light conditions or changing attentional value to the organism (pupillary responses); the ability to adapt to a constantly moving visual environemnt (waterfall effects); the ability to experience a visual object as being the same size whether near or far (size constancy); and the ability to experience the subjective visual world as stable in spite of eye movements. Specifying the mechanisms involved in these homeostatic adaptations is beyond the scope of this text and would divert from the main task. The mechanisms are reviewed in standard handbooks on vision (Davson, 1970; Graham, 1965; Jameson & Hurvich, 1972).

So far, visual homeostasis has been described either in terms of its operation upon a more general physiologic process (arousal) or in terms of its operating with certain specific visual system functions (light and dark adaptation). Little has been said about homeostatic regulation of image processing per se. Although homeostatic regulation of other specific functions indirectly contributes to the regulation of image processing, an understanding of homeostatic regulation of vision will be inadequate until it is able to account for specific regulation of image processing. However, until full details of a feedback model are described (Sec. 6.3), no basis exists for describing the regulation of image processing to be done later (Sec. 6.4).

Although I have mainly referred to homeostasis, it must not be ignored that there are also many visual mechanisms which are homeokinetic. Thus, when a resting animal visually perceives danger, visually analyzes the danger, experiences appropriate arousal and escapes, there are many kinetic shifts in many mechanisms—the resting eye becomes a moving, working eye. Iberall and McCulloch's concept (1968) will help you to understand this process.

1.12. Feedback Mechanisms in Vision

Although feedback can be assumed to play a major role in the homeostatic mechanisms just mentioned, it has not been possible in many instances to specify the properties of the involved feedback systems. There are a few instances, however, where the feedback has been thoroughly studied and the mechanisms well specified. Much of this is in the work of Stark (1968), who with his coworkers has studied the pathways and dynamic properties involved in feedback mechanisms controlling the pupil, the lens, and tracking movements. Other work in progress hopes to show the details of the pathways of feedback in fixation movements (Beeler, 1965; Fender, 1964; Weber & Daroff, 1972) and there are theories of feedback which account for the constancy of the visual world (von Holst, 1954; Matin, 1972).

Another area where feedback models have implicitly made an important contribution is in the study of receptor interaction mechanisms (Boynton, 1970; Ratliff, 1965; Werblin, 1972). As is well known, the retina is a complex of cells of different types with rich interconnections. An obvious model accounting for much happening therein is a feedback model wherein interconnections close loops. Here, however, the simple concept of feedback must be expanded to the case of many connections between many elements (a concept of networks and their properties). Network theory is the theory which attempts to explain the properties of many interconnected elements and has been used extensively in models of retinal process (Farley & Clark, 1961; Maynard, 1972; Minsky & Papert, 1969).

Many of the visual feedback mechanisms we have thus far considered are concerned with special aspects of the act of vision but might be considered as being apart from visual information processing or visual perception per se. Thus, tracking is necessary to see a moving target, but says little about how the image of the target is processed. There are several theories, however, which set for themselves the task of dealing with feedback in visual information processing. Probably the most comprehensive is that of Sokolov (1963), who shows how the adaptive processes occur internally as a result of the various sorts of information processing that take place. His work is especially striking because he can do so much with the question of visual information processing without being specific about image processing. Festinger, Burnham, Ono, and Bamber (1967), Gibson (1966), Held (1961), and Solley and Murphy (1960) all deal with perception or visual information processing but all provide theories which are either general and do not deal with psychophysiology or are dealing with specific aspects of perception other than image processing. Hebb (1949), on the other hand, has a highly physiological theory which has a concept of scanning requiring feedback control. However, his theory was developed before essential information about eye movements had been understood.

Today there would be virtual unanimity among vision scientists that a physiological understanding of perception and visual information processing must expect to rely heavily on the concept of feedback in describing specific mechanisms. It is one of the major tasks of this book to show the relationship of feedback to visual information processing.

1.13. Feedback and Nonfeedback Models
       of Visual Information Processing

One way of understanding the issue of feedback in visual information processing is to do strictly logical simple modeling between the alternatives of feedback and nonfeedback models. These can be modeled in block diagrams with a box for the eye, a box for the brain, and arrows representing channels of communication. Figure 1.7 is the nonfeedback model, with a single arrow—*from* the eye *to* the brain—while Fig. 1.8 is the feedback model with arrows in both directions.

A comparison of the two models can be made by using a further breakdown into more components. In doing so, we will use both models to account for the well-known and easily observable fact that we do not perceive everything in the environment (when we look at a given scene we sometimes see something that we had missed on an earlier occasion). Each model can account for this, but in a different way. When we use the nonfeedback model, Fig. 1.7, the eye is a passive transducer, completely dominated by the stimulation it receives. It has only one option in any situation—to send everything received, as received, to the brain. To arrive at a final percept, the brain might selectively filter what is received, but can do nothing else. The brain cannot command the eye "use optional processing method A" or "use optional processing method B," because the brain cannot "talk" to the eye. This passive method of information transmission can be called a camera-wirephoto model (Gaarder, 1963), because it shares characteristics with such a model system. A camera can only see what is there and can do so in only one way. A wirephoto transmitter can likewise only transmit what is there in the photograph from the camera and can do so in only one manner. Further, neither, of the two can be modified by the receiver.

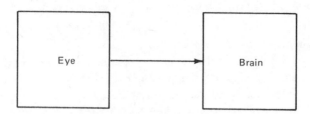

Fig. 1.7. Nonfeedback model of vision.

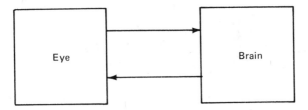

Fig. 1.8. Feedback model of vision.

Another way of considering the same issues is in terms of information. In the passive camera-wirephoto model, the receptor must always be transmitting everything impinging upon it in exactly the same way. When this constraint is applied it means that the only changes that can be made in the visual information must be made within the brain (at the lateral geniculate body or still further in). In addition, these changes can only consist of either subtracting (filtering) from the information or adding to it from other sources (distortions). This is shown in Fig. 1.9. where a visual environment is totally received and totally transmitted by the eye. A "filter" in the brain may subtract from this information. This is a nonfeedback model because there is nothing for the brain to say to the eye—the eye can only do one thing and must do it. Therefore, there could be no effect of information from the brain upon the eye. The other possibility (Fig. 1.10) is to consider that the receptor may be "set" for a particular kind of reception and transmission among several alternatives. Then, as can be seen, the information received and transmitted by the eye will already be, at any instant, a great deal less than the total amount available in the visual environment. The sizes of the arrows vividly pose the issue—between a sensory system whose first stage always transmits "everything" in the visual environment, versus a sensory system which has already at the first stage cut down on the totally available information by selecting among a number of alternatives. It is an easy step to see that the selection of alternatives must be done by the brain via a feedback. On the one hand, the law of parsimony applied to physiological considerations seems to suggest we pick the passive filter model because it appears simplest and has the fewest parts. On the other hand, the law of parsimony applied to informational considerations leads to choosing the information selector model because an adaptive sensory system receptor would not be so constructed as to receive and transmit a great deal of information about the environment that is not needed and that will be immediately filtered out at the next stage.

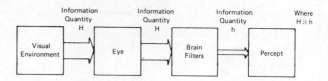

Fig. 1.9   Brain filter model of vision.

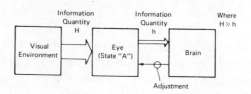

Fig. 1.10.   Feedback selector model of vision.

Thus, a further reason for favoring the idea of feedback in visual information processing. Heretofore, evidence was presented about the ubiquity of biological feedbacks, the demonstrations of the existence of feedback in special visual functions, and the need of feedback in modern theories of perception. Now the weight of the law of parsimony applied to information processing has been added.

1.14.   Analogy to the Auditory System

To this point feedback in the visual system has been considered. Now, to enhance understanding, a brief consideration of feedback in the auditory system will be made. The visual and auditory systems are the important distance receptors of animal organisms and share much in common. Likewise, in man they are the major channels for symbol perception. They have striking similarities with each other and striking differences. They are both organized around bilateral receptive organs attached to the head and they are both in close proximity to the brain with particularly large ingoing nerves connecting them with the brain. Both have small modulating muscles connected to the receptive organ and in both cases these muscles can provide a feedback channel. They each have a complex receptive organ with varieties of peripheral nerve cells and they have similar brain pathways in the geniculate bodies, colliculi, and bilateral cortical representation.

On the other hand, they deal in very different forms of sensory energy and sensory information—the electromagnetic waves of light versus the air compression of sound waves. Also, a stationary visual world is experienced much more as a three-dimensional continuum compared to the auditory world as one in which meaning is usually extracted from a temporal sequence of sounds from one or a very few sources. As a matter of fact, it is easy to see how sound is experienced as a temporal sequence, something that unfolds over time, whereas vision seems to approximate an instantaneous process.

In certain respects, the ear is an easier organ to study and for that reason was the subject of early studies on the feedback relation between a peripheral sensory receptive organ and the brain. These early studies, by Galambos, Sheatz, and Vernier, (1956), Hernandez-Peon, Scherrer and Jouvet (1956), and others were directed toward the issue of whether attention could be mediated through "gating" of input from the ear. In other words, the question was one of whether an animal can pay attention to auditory stimuli or not by "turning on" or "turning off" his ears by a message from his brain to his peripheral ear.

These experiments became classical models for the concept of feedback between the brain and a peripheral receptor and led to other experiments showing the influence of the brain on the peripheral ear.

Meticulous work by Worden, Marsh, and others, reviewed by Worden (1966) showed that the peripheral effects could be fully accounted for by other factors, such as movements of the head and external ears of the experimental animals (which are, incidently, also feedback processes in the light of further analysis; see Secs. 1.16 and 1.17). Subsequently, further work has strengthened the evidence that auditory attention is centrally controlled without peripheral gating (Picton, Hillyard, Galambos, & Schiff, 1971). However, Worden (1966) has pointed out that the evidence for feedback to the ear is very strong and that very likely the feedback plays a role in auditory perception, such as separating figure from ground in sound patterns, or in some way helping the process of "locking on" to an auditory pattern. Here, though, the investigator must await technical advances before being able to perform appropriate experiments. Comparing the auditory system with the visual system offers fresh perspectives from which to ask how feedback affects visual perception.

1.15. Defining the Visual Feedback Channels

In moving into consideration of feedback from the brain to the eye I have so far shown how the choices between feedback and nonfeedback models significantly affect information processing. The next task, using the analogy of Koch's postulates (sec. 1.9) and developing a logical case for feedback, is to attempt to demonstrate that a feedback channel is available to carry information from the brain to the eye. From logical analysis of known physiological processes, there are three ways this could be accomplished: (a) by neurohumoral processes wherein chemicals excreted by the brain would be carried to the eye through the blood stream or through other body fluids; (b) by direct neural connections, either through the optic nerve from the brain to the retina or through accessory nerves to the eye; and (c) through the musculomechanical effect of moving the eye within the socket and thereby moving the retinal image on the retina. The neurohumoral channel is of little interest in this discussion since it is the slowest acting system, operating over seconds of time or longer and therefore unable to effect the perceptual changes being studied. Neural feedbacks through accessory nerves have long been known as the feedback channel of pupil and lens mechanisms in the older literature in neurophysiology, and have been the subject of more detailed analysis recently by Stark (1968). Information transmission from the brain to the eye is taken for granted by many investigators (Sokolov, 1963); has an anatomical basis through the work of Ramon y Cajal (Polyak, 1941) and others, but has not been convincingly demonstrated in experiments involving nerve transmission. This is partly because of technical difficulties in performing the experiments, partly because of uncertainty as to what is sufficient evidence and partly because our lack of understanding of neural codes does not allow us to look for effects of optic nerve feedback upon input sensory patterning analogous to what Worden (1966) postulates in the auditory system. Although optic nerve feedback appears likely and may someday prove important, for now it must be ignored due to lack of evidence.

Thus, the brain-directed feedback of the movement of the eye in the visual world is left as the feedback whereby the effects of the brain upon the eye may be studied. This will be the issue toward which the rest of this chapter will move.

1.16. Eye Movements as Feedback

The major mechanism of feedback to be studied in this book is the mechanism of the brain causing the eye to move, which in turn causes the retinal image to move and, therefore, by changing the retinal image–retinal relationship, operates as a feedback. Figure 1.11 shows the general situation in which the retinal image of an object is moved on the retina—thus changing the retinal image–retina relation. There are a number of ways that the brain can cause the eye to move in relation to the visual environment. One is by

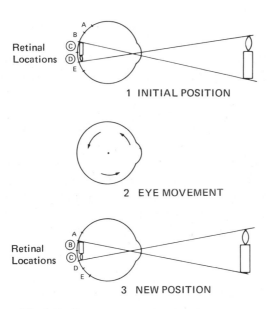

1 INITIAL POSITION

2 EYE MOVEMENT

3 NEW POSITION

Fig. 1.11. Eye movements changing the retinal image position.

moving the eye in the socket through activating the extraocular muscles. Another is by moving the head. A third is by moving the whole body and, therefore, the head, as in walking or riding. Since it is not possible to tell any great difference in the percepts under these three conditions, and to simplify the analysis, further analysis will be limited to the first case—the eye being moved in its socket by the extraocular muscles. This is not to deny the importance of the other modes, but merely to reduce the complexity of the analysis. In addition, to further simplify matters the important questions of movement of the visual environment or parts of the visual environment which are taken up by Young and Stark (1963) in their study of tracking movements will be left out of the account. Eye movements as the main feedback becomes the focus for practical study.

Studying the classification of eye movements is necessary to understand how eye movements operate as a feedback. Standard textbooks (Davson, 1970; Jameson & Hurvich, 1972) classify various types of eye movements and relate them to a variety of visual functions. These eye movements include the components of gross nystagmus, a back and forth movement of the eye in certain neurological diseases or under special conditions. Another major class of eye movement is the tracking movements the eye makes in following a target. None of these types of eye movements or their functions will be studied. Instead, consideration will be limited to large jumping fast movements the eye makes and to a finer analysis of what the eye is doing when it is apparently arresting its movement on an object of interest.

1.17. Large Eye Jumps

The two major aspects of the way the eye moves—jumping and fixating—can be readily observed. Simply observe someone's eyes as he goes about his business of adapting to his stationary environment. You will see that the eyes do essentially only two things: They *jump* with very rapid movements from one fixation to another, and they rest upon particular fixations. (A fixation is the momentary—or longer—resting of the eye at a particular position. A fixation is not necessarily looking at a particular fixation point since the external stimulus to which the eye is attending may be outside of foveal vision and may be a pattern over an area rather than a point.) The large rapid jumps from one fixation to another serve the very obvious function of allowing the more acute vision of the fovea and the near-foveal regions of the retina to be directed to the object of visual interest (Millodot, 1966). Why and how this can be considered a feedback from the brain to the eye directing visual input will be further explained in the material that follows.

These jumps of the eye are readily observed and have been extensively studied over the years. One such study has centered about the use of eye movements in the reading process, which was explored especially during the 1930s (Cunitz & Steinman, 1969; Tinker, 1958). Techniques were developed for following where the eye moved over a printed text in the reading process and a great deal was learned about the characteristics of reading eye movements. Recently, more refined techniques including those of Mackworth (1967), and Young (1963), Krauskopf (Gaarder, Silverman, Pfefferbaum, Pfefferbaum, & King, 1967) have made possible precise study of where the eye goes in its exploration of visual material such as photographs. One important limit to remember from this work is that in very rapid reading or very rapid inspection of visual material an upper limit to the rate at which the eye can jump has been found to be between four and five times a second (even though occasionally the interval between jumps may be considerably less than the 200-millisecond mean time between jumps at a rate of five times a second (see Sec. 3.3). Later text will show how this rate of jumping the eye about can be a determinant of the rate of information input of the visual system (Secs. 3.3 and 8.3).

Large eye jumps can next provide a very concrete demonstration of how eye jumps are a feedback through the mechanism of moving the retinal image on the retina.

As a very simple example which can take us to the heart of the matter, observe the brain and the eye of a college student in class. Assume that his eyes are within a visual environment providing the competing objects of a blackboard where weighty matters are made clear and a pretty girl who is pleasant to look at. Without resort to controlled experiments, assume that his brain will be telling his eyes "look here" and/or "look there." He will either look at the blackboard and deny himself the pleasure of looking at the girl, or look at the girl and not absorb what is on the board, or he will strike a compromise. The important issue is that through eye movement the brain has controlled the input from the eye and achieved a homeostatic balance (Sokolov, 1963). The visual input has been controlled by the brain by the simple mechanism of looking at one place rather than another. Eye movements are part of the feedback chain that accomplishes this. This is a feedback mechanism because what is originally on the retinal image is analyzed and the result of that analysis is used to determine what shall next be on the retinal image through the use of eye movements to change the direction of looking. This forms a chain of events in the perceptual act as follows: (1) original retinal image; (2) transmission of this retinal image to the brain; (3) analysis of the retinal image by the brain and decision as to where to look next; and (4) movement of the eye to a new scene with a new retinal image (Fig. 1.12).

A number of models of visual perception are particularly concerned with large eye jumps as a major element in the act of visual perception. In particular, Festinger et al. (1967) and Festinger (1971) consider the efference of eye movements as a necessary component of the visual act and Hochberg (1964) uses the analogy of pointing a television camera. Luriia, Pradvina-Vinarskaia, and Yarbus (1961) and Thomas (1968) have similar models.

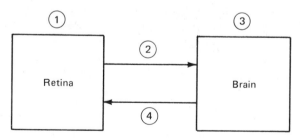

Fig. 1.12. Chain of events in eye movement feedback.

1.18. Small Fixation Eye Jumps

When you observe someone's eye jumping about, you will notice that if you will ask the person to stop looking about and stare at a point that his eye apparently stops moving. This is the fixation referred to above. Even if you look very closely at the person's eye while he is fixating for many seconds you probably will not see any motion. If the person has reasonably good control over his eyes he should be able to maintain his fixation with no apparent motion for several minutes and perhaps for as long as he wishes. Superficially, he will also not notice any gross changes in his vision when he does this, although if he is a more careful observer he will notice the loss of detail of his peripheral vision and slight changes of the percept. The apparent fact that this motionless eye can maintain good vision for as long as wished might be taken as putting to an end the idea of feedback in visual as a crucial necessity, since if there is no feedback motion and yet vision continues, then obviously the feedback is unnecessary.

For this reason, feedback models of the visual process which had eye movements as a crucial cause of feedback from the changed retinal image could be easily dismissed. One of the earliest such models was that of Marshall and Talbot (1942), wherein the acuity of vision was assumed to be sharpened by the movement of the retinal image over receptors due to slight tremor of the eye. This model has subsequently been shown deficient by many studies (see Steinman, Haddad, Skavenski, & Wyman 1973), but will probably someday be recognized in the same light as the efferent gating models of the auditory system—a pioneering study incorrect in specific details but containing a kernel of new insight hitherto ignored (Worden, 1966).

A feedback model with eye movements causing retinal image feedback is heavily dependent upon the nature of eye movements during long fixations. Therefore, it was of crucial importance when fixation eye movements were accurately measured for the first time during the early 1950s. These studies showed that contrary to appearance at gross visual inspection, the eye continues to move even during fixation (Fig. 1.13). Even though earlier work had hinted this was the case, much better measuring techniques were required to show unequivocally that motion was always present in the eye. The improved technique involved reflecting light from a small mirror attached to a tight-fitting contact lens worn on the eye. The reflected light formed an "optical lever" that amplified the movements of the eye for recording purposes. Thus the technical barriers to measurements of these eye movements were solved. As is often the case in scientific discovery, this work

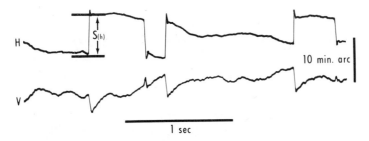

Fig. 1.13. Fixation eye movements. Recorded by the contact lens technique. Time moves from left to right. H is horizontal component, V is vertical component of eye movement. Eye jumps are readily seen; S(h) is a specific example marked in the horizontal record. Drift especially evident in vertical record after eye jumps. Tremor most easily seen in vertical record. (From "Fine Eye Movements During Inattention" by K. Gaarder, *Nature,* 1966, **209**, 83. Reprinted by permission of the editor.)

was carried out independently in at least three different laboratories at about the same time—in England (Ditchburn & Ginsborg, 1953), the Soviet Union (Yarbus, 1967), and the United States (Riggs, Armington, & Ratliff, 1954). The most important fact about fixation eye movements discovered in this work was that the rapid jumps of the eye are still present, even though the eye is apparently fixated. The reason the rapid jumps cannot be seen is because they are too small. They are of a size of about 10 minutes of arc (1/6 of a degree of arc on the globe of the eye) or less, which is less than 0.01 inch of movement on the surface of the eye and less than the diameter of 30 cone receptors. In addition to the continuing eye jumps, that occur about once a second, there are also other components to the fixation eye movements: slow drifting of the eye and a rapid small oscillation of the eye of much smaller amplitude (about 0.5 minute of arc) termed "tremor." These other movements will not presently be considered because to do so would divert the main direction of arguments concerning the eye jumps. (The eye jumps, incidentally, are often called "saccades" in the scientific literature. While the term is widely used by specialists, the fact that nonspecialists are generally unacquainted with it points to the desirability of using the more straightforward term "jump" from English rather than this obscure French word, which means to jerk on the reins of a horse. Other terms for eye jumps are eye "jerks" and "flicks.") Later (Sec. 6.5) we will consider the recent experiments of Steinman et al. (1973) and others, reporting long periods of fixation without eye jumps, when we consider objections to a feedback model of vision.

1.19. Eye Jumps as the Particular Feedback

At this point let me recapitulate the central fact that both in normal vision over a large visual scene and fixation on a smaller part of the visual world, the eye is almost always and inevitably making rapid jumps, often as frequently as four times a second, but rarely less than once every few seconds. Because any eye movement shifts the retinal image on the retina and thereby changes the eye and its stimulus, these jumps represent a feedback from the brain (which commands) to the eye (the organ of visual reception).

Even if this is accepted as a logical fact, since the movements of the eye fulfill the logical criteria necessary to establish a feedback, it remains to be shown that eye movements do actually function as a feedback. We have now reached the point of departure from known fact and logic and it is necessary to use experimentation to allow further analysis of the problem. Without such experimentation it could be argued that even though a feedback exists, there is no reason to assume it has any crucial role in visual perception—that it is merely an epiphenomenon that keeps the eye on target but is otherwise irrelevant.

EXPERIMENTALLY DEMONSTRATING FEEDBACK IN VISION

1.20. Rationale

From what has been said up until now, some of the elements to be considered in an experiment to demonstrate feedback in visual perception have become clearer. First, it is necessary to use eye movement as the channel of feedback to be examined, since it can be readily catalogued as a hypothetical connection and is technically measurable. Second, since the presence of feedback in large eye jumps is self-evident and since demonstration of feedback in large eye jumps would not prove feedback present in small eye jumps, there is more merit in using small eye jumps as the specific manifestation of feedback to be examined. Third, since horizontal and vertical eye jumps manifest themselves by changes of the position of the retinal image upon the visual plane, stimuli which differ in their orientation on the visual plane seem the logical ones to use (Fig. 1.14).

Thus, one useful experimental approach would consist of presenting a particular visual stimulus in various orientations within the visual plane while the subject's fixation eye jumps are examined. The general rationale of this experiment can be made still more explicit in schematic diagrams. In Fig. 1.15 two different conditions of visual stimulation are shown—with visual

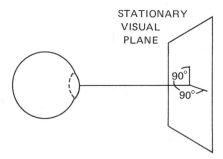

Fig. 1.14. Schematic diagram of the stationary visual plane relative to the eye.

display (or stimulus) A and with visual display B. According to what has been proposed above, the expectation is "that at any given instant in the perceptual act the perceptual system has used the data taken in so as to be able to change the state of the receptor suitably for taking in the next increment of data. This implies that if the stimulus changes then the cumulative centrifugal actions taken would change" (Gaarder, 1960 p. 471; see also Sokolov 1963, pp. 5-6). Considering Fig. 1.15 at any instant, you would say that stimulus A will have produced an "A state" in the eye, resulting in the transmission of A information over the optic nerve; this will cause an A state in the brain, and that A state will cause A movements of the extraocular muscles, resulting in a further A change on the retina of the eye adaptively modifying the A state of the eye. Stimulus B would likewise cause its unique changes in the same chain. Taking Fig. 1.15 over a period of time, it can be said that a period of viewing stimulus A would have caused the eye to be in a set of A states which would have caused the transmission of sets of A information to the brain, causing a set of A states in the brain, which in turn caused a set of A movements of the extraocular muscles. Finally, these "A movements" would cause "A changes" on the retina, and because this is a feedback system, those "A changes" would be one of the determinants of the set of the "A states" of the eye. There is a cycle involved since it is a circular chain of causality.

From this, an experimental hypothesis may be derived that if appropriately different stimuli are presented to the eye, there will be cumulatively different eye movements for each different stimulus. In other words, if the eye looks at different stimuli, somehow the movements of the eye ought to be different. If this is found to be the case, a still further assumption is necessary to justify the idea of feedback. This assumption is that the different

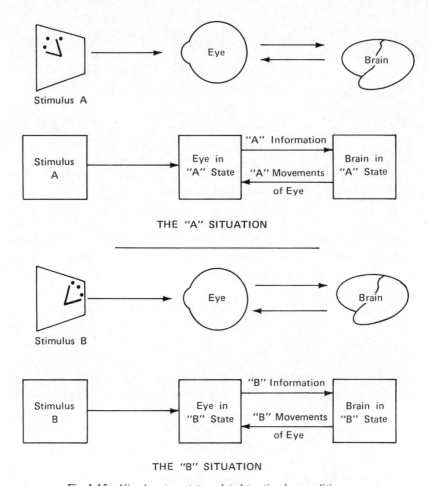

Fig. 1.15. Visual system states related to stimulus conditions.

resultant eye movements of different stimuli do in fact have an important role in modifying the retinal image, the information transmitted over the optic nerve, and the evolving percept in the brain. To some, this will be self-evident from what has already been said; for others, the concrete demonstrations of the effects of different eye movements on the retinal image may help to bridge the gap. This is done in Chap. 4 (Secs. 4.6 and 4.8) where photographic simulations show these same effects.

Since the search is for a feedback in small fixation eye movement, which causes dislocations of the eye relative to the stationary visual plane, it is important to visualize the movements of the eye relative to this visual plane.

(The stationary visual plane, Fig. 1.14, can be thought of as an imaginary screen in front of the eyes during fixation which is perpendicular to the major line of sight upon which the objects of the visual environment can be projected.) It is evident, therefore, that one of the things about which the most information is possessed is eye movement relative to the visual plane. Therefore, the different stimuli which have the best chance of showing such different movements might be expected to be those that differed mainly in the orientation of the stimuli within the visual plane. It was for this reason that a particular type of stimulus would be chosen (Fig. 1.16). As can be seen, there is a pattern with a part of it coming to a point at the center of the visual field. The pattern can be presented in any of the four quadrants about the center of the display. The important thing to notice about the particular combination of stimulus variables and dependent eye movement variables is that analogous changes are possible in the eye movements matching the changes in the visual stimulus—i.e., horizontal and vertical orientational changes of the simulus can be matched by horizontal and vertical changes of the eye movements.

This experimental design tests the idea that feedback, manifested by small eye jumps controlling retinal image movement, may influence visual perception. If eye jumps have no relation to the stimulus orientation, there is no reason to assume that feedback operates. On the other hand, if eye jumps are affected by the stimulus orientation, as predicted by the feedback model, this is presumptive evidence for feedback.

1.21. Experimental Demonstration of the Relationship between Visual Stimulus Orientation and Fixation Eye Jumps

One experimental demonstration consists of measuring a subject's fixation eye movements while he fixates upon the stimuius (Fig. 1.16) in each of its four orientational positions. In an experiment that I reported elsewhere (Gaarder, 1960), five experimental runs of 45 seconds were done in each of the four positions and then the mean eye jump was computed for each run after measuring each eye jump individually.

Figure 1.17 shows the mean eye jumps (i.e., the mean saccades) for each of the four quadrants. The five runs for each position are represented by the five connected points. The striking thing this experiment shows is that changing the position of the stimulus within the visual display from one quadrant to another caused a similar but opposite change in the mean eye jumps occuring during that run. This is predicted in the hypothetical model of the situation—that a change in the stimulus should cause a change in the feedback which controls the input of the information from the stimulus by the receptor.

This can be considered strong presumptive evidence favoring the general hypothesis that changing the stimulus changes the eye movements which change the retinal image and, therefore, changes the way the information is taken in, so that "if the stimulus changes then the cumulative centrifugal actions taken would change" (Gaarder, 1960, p. 471). Another set of experiments testing the same hypothesis provided the same results (Gaarder, 1967a). Work of Steinman (1965), undertaken for other reasons, is also consistent with the hypothesis, because he concluded that retinal "local sign"

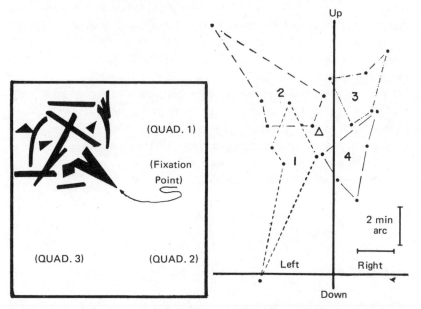

Fig. 1.16. Visual stimulus with four possible orientations in the visual plane. The stimulus in in Quadrant 4 in this diagram. The fixation is always at the center of the field.

Fig. 1.17. Eye jumps under different stimulus conditions. Distribution of the mean eye jumps of the four positions. Dotted lines connect the five mean eye jumps of the same quadrant. Quadrant indicated by number, grand mean of means by Δ.

(From "Relating a Component of Physiological Nystagmus to Visual Display" by K. Gaarder, *Science*, August 1960, **132**, 471–472. Copyright 1960 by the American Association for the Advancement of Science.)

was a stimulus for corrective eye jumps. Herman, working with Nachmias, has also found these results (unpublished experiments).

1.22. Recapitulation

It has been shown how feedback is a concrete physiological mechanism underlying homeostatic and adaptive processes. Various principles of feedback in living and nonliving systems have been reviewed as a basis for studying feedback in the visual system. The many feedbacks operative in the visual system have been considered, with particular emphasis upon the question of a role for feedback in visual perception. The case of vision during fixation upon a stimulus was analyzed. It was shown logically how the movement of the eyes, which changes the way the visual stimulus impinges on the retinal image, is a feedback linkage. Finally, it was shown experimentally that changing the visual stimulus changes the pattern of eye movements, which in turn must have the circular effect of changing the next increment of new visual input. This is strong evidence for feedback playing an important role in visual perception and provides a foundation for a model of visual perception to emerge later (Chaps. 4 & 6).

2
EVOKING RESPONSES WITH THE EYE JUMP AS TRIGGER

2.1. Introduction

In this chapter further experimental observations will be accumulated, based on the use of a new computing technique. Out of this will come one reason for considering a special conception of time relationships within the visual system. Instead of the implicit, common sense idea of visual information processing being of a continuous, analog nature, consider the idea that eye jumps break up visual information processing into discrete, discontinuous quantal units.

The route to this insight will combine three disparate ideas. The first of these—feedback—was introduced in Chap. 1; its essence is that the brain has an effect upon vision by moving the eye in a determinate patterned way through eye jumps. The second idea—the specific discrete response by an organism to a specific discrete stimulus—is embodied concretely in the evoked response of classical neurophysiology and, by extension, in the averaged evoked response recorded by the computer of averaged transients (CAT) (see Sec. 2.2). The third idea—discrete, discontinuous step functions (Sec. 2.3)—is the crucial means of linking these other two ideas. Instead of an external discrete event triggering an internal response, the idea of internal triggering by the discrete event of an eye jump must be assimilated. What will emerge in Chaps. 4 and 6 is that a feedback event—the eye jump—is a discrete, discontinuous triggering event resulting in the discontinuous generation and transmission of information to the brain.

In order to understand these ideas, begin by examining simple details of how the CAT averages evoked responses (Sec. 2.2). After that will come the first step toward understanding discontinuity by describing discrete step functions (Sec. 2.3). I will then show a specific experiment using eye jumps as the trigger of the CAT (Secs. 2.4 & 2.5). Other experiments using the same basic idea will add weight to the idea (Sec. 2.6) and other interpretations of the same experiment will be considered (Sec. 2.7). Finally, the ideas of the chapter will be recapitulated (Sec. 2.8).

2.2. The Computer of Averaged Transients

In classical neurophysiology the prototypical experiment takes the form of using microelectrodes to record brain activity from a specific site—either a single cell or the cells in a particular location—while a specific stimulus is applied somewhere to the organism. The stimulus can either be applied to an intact receptor system or to parts of the organism directly, such as shocking a nerve or another brain site. Out of thousands of these experiments has evolved an implicit doctrine—that the scientific principle of determinism applies to animal nervous systems in the form of specific stimuli eliciting specific responses. Part of the specificity of response is that responses often have highly regular relationships to stimuli in such properties as the temporal course of the response, the size of the response, and the specific anatomical-functional location of the response. In the visual system such work has shown that visual stimuli produce single cell responses and responses of groups of cells in the cell layers of the retina, the fibers of the optic nerve and optic radiations, the lateral geniculate body and the visual cortex, to mention some of the most important sites.

However, these classical experiments can only be carried out in surgically prepared animals or humans undergoing brain surgery for other reasons. Therefore, the development of techniques that made it possible to record such responses to stimuli in the intact animal or human was of great significance.

At first the technique was itself laborious and required hours of technical work to be utilized. Then in the early 1960s, as computers were more widely available it became possible to use this technique with a computer doing all the tedious calculations very rapidly. Although a general purpose computer could be programmed to make the calculations, a special purpose computer was designed whose main function was to make these calculations automatically. This was the computer of averaged transients.

We may understand its place by considering the dilemma confronting the experimenter evaluating an animal or human in a test situation. Suppose a particular low intensity stimulus such as a flash of light or a click is presented to a subject 100 times while his brain waves are being recorded. Ordinarily, an experimenter would be unable to examine the record of the subject's brain waves and see any evidence of the stimulation in the recording. Yet the principle of determinism demands clearly that somehow the stimulus (cause) must have some response (effect) in the brain. We can simply explain why no such effect is seen by saying it is because there is so much "noise" in the brain waves that the response is lost. That is to say, the brain manifests electrical activity reflecting so many other operations, irrelevant to the processing of the stimulus, resulting in other brain waves unrelated to it, that the response to the stimulus is lost among these other activities. Thus other activities represent "noise" relative to the crucial cause and effect operation we are trying to observe. The progress of classical neurophysiology was made because this problem was not present to the same degree. By using experimental subjects (usually animals) where electrodes could be implanted in the substance of the brain at the precise location desired it was possible to obtain localized responses that were relatively uncontaminated by irrelevant activity. Thus, in the situation where the experimenter cannot open the skull of the subject, he knows from earlier work that something is happening in the subject's brain but he can't get at it and study it. It is here that the averaging technique solves some of the investigator's problems, and I will now briefly show how this is done.

By way of explanation, I use an analogy between ocean waves and brain waves (Fig. 2.1). This analogy is very precise in many formal respects, so one may move interchangeably back and forth between considering brain waves and ocean waves. Assume that along some particular ocean pier you are able to drop identical small pebbles into the water at a particular location. Also assume that you are able to record accurately the water level at a spot 6 inches away. This is analogous to neurophysiological experiments. The pebbles represent stimuli and the recorded waves represent responses. On a calm day the pebbles would cause definite repetitive predictable waves to be recorded at the recording site. Each recorded wave would be quite similar to the next. This is the analogy to the experiment of the early neurophysiologist who places his electrodes at the appropriate quiet recording site. Next, imagine a stormy day when the water is splashing about. If the experiment is performed again, on examining the record of waves from the recording site, the investigator will be unable to tell when a pebble was dropped. And yet,

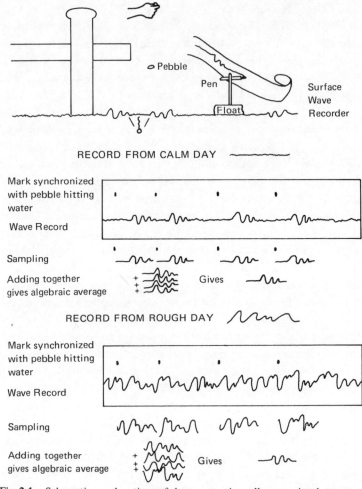

Fig. 2.1. Schematic explanation of how averaging allows a signal to appear through noise. The analogy is used of a pebble dropped in water causing waves which are recorded on a strip chart. See text for a description of how samples are added to cancel out the noise in the record.

scientific view leaves no doubt that the fact the pebble dropped is manifested in the record, if only we knew how to extract the information. It has been buried in the noise of the extraneous activity. This is analogous to the plight of the experimenter recording brain waves through the scalp and, again the dilemma is before us.

The way the information is extracted is by averaging the wave activities following the stimulus events. Assume that each time the pebble strikes the water a synchronizing signal (trigger) is given to the recorder and the next 3 seconds of wave activity are sampled and suitably stored. After a series of stimuli giving a series of synchronizing signals, there would be stored a series of samples of wave activity following the stimuli. It is relatively simple for a computer to add the signals together algebraically point for point along the horizontal (time) dimension of the wave. When this is done one has the "average" wave for the period in question. Since the "noise" of the irrelevant activity is random relative to the stimuli, it averages out to near zero, whereas the buried response becomes visible in the record. This is the basic principle of response averaging—activity following a synchronizing signal produced by the stimulus is serially averaged so that the random noise of the signal is eliminated by averaging and the buried response becomes visible. This is diagrammed in Fig. 2.1. There can be seen the contrast between a noiseless and a noisy recording situation. The drop of the pebble in the water defines the synchronizing signal (the analog of the external stimulus). The raw record is then automatically broken into samples as it is generated and the samples are algebraically summed by the computer. (An actual illustration of this with brain waves is shown in Chap. 3 in Fig. 3.4.)

The basic idea this experimental procedure makes tangible is the implicit doctrine of classical neurophysiology referred to at the beginning of this section—that a known stimulus causes a specific definitive response whose characteristics over time are measurable. Although the averaging technique has the major advantage of being usable with the intact experimental animal or human, it does not have the fine-grained accuracy of microelectrode techniques. Especially, it is difficult to localize accurately responses to definite anatomical-functional areas and it is not practical to isolate individual nerve spike firing from the response. Likewise, the averaged response is the average of many responses to many stimuli and does not necessarily represent any one response. On the other hand, as evidence accumulates, it is being found that averaged responses from the scalp are highly correlated with direct wave recordings and with individual cell recordings (Creutzfeldt, Watanabe, & Lux, 1966; Fox & O'Brien, 1965; Pollen, Lee, & Taylor, 1971). In addition, there are correlations with information delivery (Sutton, Tueting, Zubin, & John, 1967), stimulus form (John, Herrington, & Sutton, 1967), stimulus properties (Ruchkin & John, 1966), stimulus meaning (Chapman, 1973), and hemispheric localization (Biersdorf & Nakamura, 1971; Cohn, 1971).

2.3. Discrete Discontinuous Step Functions

Next to consider is the gap between what we have just discussed—averaging responses with the CAT—and the contents of the first chapter—eye jumps as a feedback in the visual process. The common denominator in each of these is the occurrence of an abrupt discrete event. In the case of the averaging technique, the discrete event is the occurrence of the stimulus which triggers the synchronized signal starting the averaging sampling of the computer. In the case of the visual process, the discrete event is the jump of the eye. This can also be discussed as a manifestation of another biomechanical process—a step function. Ashby has provided a good discussion of step functions, which he defines as variables having "finite intervals of constancy separated by instantaneous jumps" (Ashby, 1960, pp. 87–99). A common sense conception of a step function is that it is any variable whose method of change is to make abrupt discrete incremental jumps rather than to change smoothly and continuously (Fig. 2.2).

By recognizing the fact that an eye jump presents an abrupt discrete jump, we may see an analogy between it and the abrupt onset of an external stimulus and thereby have before us the possibility of using the eye jump as the triggering or synchronizing stimulus for the CAT. To understand the experiment this suggests, it is very important to grasp the points that have just been made: The CAT uses a trigger signal that is synchronous with an event—which is usually the presentation of an external stimulus—as a means to activate the computer for taking a sample of internal activity following that event. By repetition of the event, repeated samples are collected and averaged. Thereby a response may be seen which would otherwise be buried in noise. The usual synchronous event which triggers the computer is the presentation of an external stimulus. However, this procedure is being modified here in a unique way: using the jump of the eye as the synchronizing event triggering the CAT. Thus, instead of measuring the response to an external stimulus, the response to an internal event of the

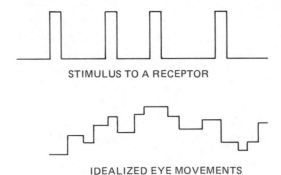

STIMULUS TO A RECEPTOR

IDEALIZED EYE MOVEMENTS

Fig. 2.2. Examples of step functions.

organism is being measured; you learned in Chap. 1 (Secs. 1.16-1.19), that this response also causes an abrupt change in the retinal image. In later chapters (Secs. 3.2, 4.2, 4.3, 5.6, & 7.2), further elaboration of the idea of discontinuity will be made and further implications explored. Next is a description of the experiment suggested by these ideas.

2.4. The Concept of the Experiment

From the material just presented, one can derive a specific experiment: a subject can view an unchanging stimulus while his fixation eye movements are recorded. At the same time the brain waves from the occipital scalp can be recorded from surface electrodes. The occipital area is at the back of the head and lies over that part of the cerebral cortex which is associated with vision. Each time the subject's eye jumps, a trigger signal is gotten by electronically processing the electrical derivative of his eye movement. The trigger signal, which is caused by, and synchronized with his eye movement, is then used to trigger the computer of averaged transients. The computer then samples the brain activity that follows and averages a number of the samples. One has thereby measured the average activity of the visual cortex following the jump of the eye (Gaarder, Krauskopf, Graf, Kropfl, & Armington, 1964).

2.5. Experimental Demonstration of Eye Jump
Linked Evoked Responses

The form of the experiment was summarized in Sec. 2.4. To enable greater understanding, the experiment will be described in greater detail. The question the experiment will answer positively is: Does the jump of the eyes, which can be precisely caught as a moment of time, cause the transmission of a burst of nerve impulse (and consequently information) to the visual cortex? More details of recording fixation eye movements are described elsewhere (Gaarder et al., 1967). The subject fixates a stimulus which consists of an illuminated spot 20 minutes of arc in diameter (1/3 of a degree of arc). Brain waves are recorded by a standard technique—one electrode is placed on the inion, the bony prominence at the back of the skull, lying over the occipital cerebral cortex and the other electrode is placed 2 inches above it, so that between the two electrodes one picks up brain activity representing part of the activity in the visual cerebral cortex, which is in the occipital area.

An eye movement trigger circuit is set so that it will discriminate eye jumps, immediately putting out a trigger pulse for each jump (see also Sec. 7.5). This in turn triggers the CAT, which takes the next 1/2 second of EEG

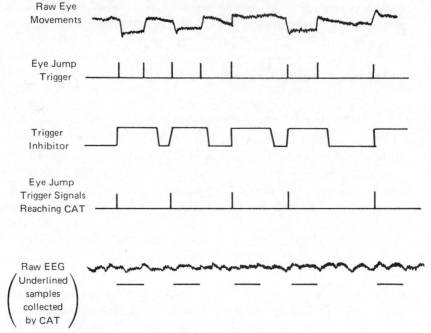

Fig. 2.3. Schematic explanation of averaging brain activity following eye jumps. Top trace (raw eye movements) is the raw record of the eye movements with the eye jumps easily seen. The next trace (eye jump trigger) shows the output of a trigger set to give pulses whenever an eye jump occurs. The third trace (trigger inhibitor) operates for over 0.5 second each time an eye jump registers to prevent further eye jumps from registering for at least 0.5 second. The fourth trace (eye jump trigger signals reaching CAT) shows the effect of the trigger inhibitor in blocking out many eye jump triggerings to avoid triggering the CAT before a sample is collected. The last trace (raw EEG) has the samples collected by the CAT underlined. These samples are averaged by the CAT to give an evoked response linked to the eye jumps (see Fig. 3.4 for an example).

to store. Figure 2.3 shows this schematically in a simulated sample of record. As explained above (Sec. 2.2), each sample collected by the CAT contains a "signal" buried in the "noise" of the sample and by collecting a number of samples, this signal is averaged out to appear in the tracing.

The result of the experiment is to show that the jump of the eye is followed by brain activity in the occipital (visual) cerebral cortex which is indistinguishable from that caused by a flashing light under other experimental conditions. If it is assumed that these brain waves reflect the transmission of information to the visual cortex (Sutton et al., 1967), then it has been shown that the input of visual information occurs in "bursts" related to and following eye jumps.

2.6. Verification of the Eye Jump Linked Evoked Response

The idea of brain wave changes related to eye jumps first emerged during the early 1950s in the concept of lambda waves—grossly visible brain waves most prominent in the occipital area, felt to be an oculomotor system response (Bickford & Klass, 1964). These are obviously the same phenomena as the eye jump linked evoked response, which has been sharpened by the averaging technique. In addition, numerous studies have now invariably found eye jump linked evoked responses, both with fine eye movement eye jumps and larger eye jumps (Armington, Gaarder, & Schick, 1967; Barlow, 1964; Gaarder, 1968; Remond, Lesevre, & Torres, 1965; Scott & Bickford, 1967). In studying large eye jumps the nature of the response is related to the eye jump in the following ways: (a) The evoked response to large eye jumps is dependent on the distance that the eye jumps, with the general nature being that the further the eye jumps the larger the response. (b) The evoked response to the eye jumping from left to right is different than the evoked response to the eye jumping from right to left. (c) The evoked response to the eye jump depends on the nature of the visual scene or stimulus across which it jumps. (d) It is possible to differentiate an "on" evoked response (jumping across a boundary from dark to light) from an "off" evoked response (jumping across a boundary from light to dark) (Gaarder, 1968). These descriptions can be better understood by referring to Fig. 4.3 in Chap. 4. By generalizing, it may be said that the experiments show the nature of the response in the visual cortex to eye jumps is related to the nature of the visual stimulus and to the nature of the subject's orientation within the visual environment.

In other experiments, not only has the occipital response been measured, but averaged electroretinograms were also recorded and found to be detectable and related to the nature of the stimulus (Armington et al., 1967), showing directly that there is measurable change of the retina associated with eye jumps.

2.7. Other Interpretations

The usual interpretation of the results of occipital visual evoked response studies is that these responses reflect the transmission to the visual cortex of information about the visual image. The studies reported herein go a step further and use the eye jump as a trigger for averaging rather than using the onset of an external stimulus, and it is concluded that the meaning of the response is the same. There are other possible interpretations of the facts that can be examined at this point:

1. *Occipital evoked responses to visual stimuli represent something other than neural activity of the visual cortex.* This argument has been advanced by Bickford, Jacobson, and Cody (1964) and others on the assumption that the recorded activity represents muscle action potentials or some other source of electrical activity. Aside from the difficulty entailed in hypothesizing muscle activity with onset latencies much shorter than known, this interpretation has not withstood experimental examination where it has been shown that there is a high degree of correlation between cortical nerve spike firing, cortical brain wave activity from the nearby area and the overlying scalp wave activity (Creutzfeldt et al., 1966; Fox & O'Brien, 1965; Pollen et al., 1971). The only parsimonious way of explaining this congruence is to assume evoked responses reflect the firing of neurons.

2. *Eye jump linked occipital evoked responses are related to eye muscle regulation rather than image processing.* This interpretation cannot be sustained for several reasons: (*a*) The form of the evoked responses has been shown to be the same as the form of evoked responses to externally changed stimuli when eye movements are not present (Gaarder et al., 1964). (*b*) The form of the evoked response is highly correlated with a number of properties of the constant stimulus, such as intensity and form (Gaarder, 1968), in a way which overrides the relationship between the response and the size of the eye jumps. (*c*) Animal study has shown that the evoked response to eye movements can be elicited all along the visual pathway—at the optic chiasm, optic tract, lateral geniculate body and visual cortex (Rhodes, Lanoir, Saier, & Naquet, 1962). Nothing but visual responses are felt to travel this pathway. (*d*) There is no detectable response other than alpha-locking before the onset of the eye jump, although some formed activity would be expected if the occipital response controlled eye movements (Gaarder, Koresco, & Kropfl, 1966b). (*e*) Although there are instances in which the evoked response is larger with larger eye movements, there are also instances in which it is smaller (Gaarder, 1968, see Fig. 5, p. 696). This fits with the idea of a change related to the net change of retinal area stimulation but not with the idea of a change related primarily to the size of the eye movement.

3. *Evoked responses are recorded over the entire scalp to any stimulus in any sense modality and are therefore nonspecific.* The specificity of the evoked response is demonstrated within the context of differentiation in a single experiment. The fact responses are found everywhere is accountable by assuming, as do many neurophysiologists (Sokolov, 1963, p. 261), that stimuli *are* registered over most of the cerebral cortex even though their primary processing is done in restricted locations.

4. *Eye jump linked evoked responses are representations of mechanisms for maintaining the constancy of the visual world or for accommodating to the retinal "smear" produced by eye jumps.* This interpretation is quite compatible with the interpretation being offered herein, and therefore does not affect it either way.

5. *Even though brain waves responses occur, this does not mean visual information is transmitted.* This argument not only ignores the specificity of evoked responses, but also ignores the law of parsimony by postulating a great deal of useless activity. In fairness to both sides of the interpretations, it is best to remember that these questions cannot yet be considered settled and that we must remain open to the consideration of new evidence. Further alternative interpretations and criticisms of the model will be presented later (Sec. 6.5).

2.8. Recapitulation

In Chap. 1 I showed how eye movements could be conceptualized as a feedback in the visual perceptual process and how vision could be shown to be related to that feedback. In the present chapter more has been made of the fact that it is the eye jumps, occurring periodically and representing discontinuities or step functions in the perceptual process, which are of major importance. This means, combining the two central themes of feedback and of discontinuity, that the brain somehow controls visual input and that it does so not by a continuous (analog) adjustment of the eye, but by intermittently or discontinuously making movements that result in abruptly new retinal image configurations being presented to the brain, as reflected by the occurrence of typical visual evoked responses over the visual cortex. Although the same conclusions could be reached by strictly logical analysis of the known facts (see Gaarder, 1966c), the demonstration of an eye jumped linked response adds weight to the conclusion.

So far, my two main methods have been those of using a new theoretical entity (feedback) as a predictor of experimental results and of using analogy between the step function of eye jumps and the step function trigger of a new experimental technique. This is not a major synthesis of a model of the visual process. A further task will be to show how such a model can be elaborated (Chap. 4), mainly using the two concepts already developed—feedback and discontinuity. Before doing this, however, I shall explore further an issue in psychophysiology that has been implied but has not yet been specified. This is the issue of cortical excitability cycles or of central intermittency, which will be discussed in Chap. 3 and related to eye jumps. After having assimilated this third factor, our model can be built.

3 RELATIONS BETWEEN INTRINSIC BRAIN CYCLES AND EYE JUMPS

3.1. Introduction

This chapter will deal with a number of issues that further clarify the question of discontinuity in brain functions introduced in Chap. 2. These issues may be introduced around the elusive concept of periodicity in brain functions which has occupied neurophysiologists since the end of the last century. Periodicity may properly be viewed as only one aspect of the temporal structure of events, to be studied later in greater detail (Chaps. 6-8). Ashby (1960, 1963) has emphasized in his penetrating studies how much may be achieved by the serial temporal analysis of various events. When an event recurs regularly at predictable time intervals, it may be considered periodic and it may also be considered cyclical. Periodicity is a clue that signals the investigator to seek further understanding of relationships leading to its occurrence. On the other hand, temporal analysis often shows the regular recurrence of an event or a chain of events without the intervening time intervals exhibiting exact periodicity. These recurrences may then be considered cycles; this being the more general case.

A cycle may, for our purposes, be conveniently defined as a set of events tending to recur in a similar sequence under similar conditions. The broader definition includes periodicity, but also includes cycles which differ somewhat in the elements of the cycle, in the time to complete an elemental step of the cycle and in the sequencing of the elements of the cycle. Therefore, the times to complete cycles need not be identical, so that strict periodicity need not occur.

In the investigation of the brain, many solid studies point toward periodicity without much coherence as to underlying meaning and mechanisms. As a result, neurophysiologists are of divided opinions—some tentatively accept the idea of periodicity in the brain and struggle with the task of elucidating its nature, while others find the evidence insufficient to warrant serious consideration and, therefore, ignore the issue. Although the idea has not been refuted, it must be acknowledged that it has neither been possible to arrive at a concrete understanding of the mechanisms underlying periodicity nor to do more than demonstrate its occurrence in specific instances while failing to demonstrate its general role in brain function. Excellent reviews by Bertelson (1966), Harter (1967), and White (1963) can introduce the reader to the detailed arguments concerning the idea of periodicity. White observes precursors of the idea in the work of Henri Bergson and William James. Also, Poggio and Viernstein (1964) have shown periodicity in many thalamic sensory neuron sequences. The particular aspect of periodicity we are interested in has to do with the brain being more receptive to stimuli at one moment than the next and of its operating, therefore, in very rapid short cycles.

In the next section (Sec. 3.2), we will examine further a question closely related to periodicity—that of continuity versus discontinuity—looked at earlier. Periodicity may involve either continuous or discontinuous functions, and we will favor the idea of discontinuity. In Sec. 3.3, we will then consider alpha rhythm, the major tangible manifestation of periodicity in the brain. Section 3.4 will provide evidence for a major manifestation of periodicity in a precise relation between alpha and beta rhythms. Periodicity in eye jumps (Sec. 3.5) will then be examined and in Sec. 3.6 we will describe how eye jumps are related to alpha rhythm. We are then in a position to recapitulate the issues around periodicity (Sec. 3.7) and prepare to consider in Chap. 4 how a model can be synthesized.

3.2. Continuity versus Discontinuity in Brain Functioning

In the previous chapter we showed how consideration of the nature of eye jumps led to using the concept of discontinuity, as manifested in the step function of eye jumps (Sec. 2.3). Here we will take up the analogous problem of continuity versus discontinuity in the brain in relation to how the brain processes information over time. These issues will then be discussed further when we consider the model of discontinuous visual information processing in Chap. 4. In looking at the class of discontinuous phenomena, we can see that a variety of terms can be used to describe them. Each of these terms has its own nuances of meaning and may have a technical definition in its usage in a certain field or may even have several definitions in several fields. The terms that follow share the idea of discontinuity: packages and packaging, samples and sampling, gating, chopped and chopping, incremental, chunks and chunking, intermittent, periodic, cyclical, rhythmic, quantal, psychological moments, psychological units of duration, central scanning, excitability cycles, neuronic shutters. Each of these terms has been used by some physiologists and psychologists to explain a range of things they have studied. Since each has slightly different meanings, it will remain for further work to clarify an appropriate conceptual framework to consolidate the data and ideas involved.

As a further complication, it must be noted that periodic phenomena are not necessarily intrinsically discontinuous, but may sometimes rightly be considered continuous. The waxing and waning of sea tides is an example of a continuous function, in contrast to the release of a clockwork escapement mechanism by a pendulum swinging or the steps of unlocking a combination lock which are discontinuous. However, all the phenomena which we will consider—nerve spikes, eye jumps, etc.—are of a discontinuous nature and it will be with discontinuity that we are concerned.

3.3. Alpha Rhythm

It might appear that some sort of regularity in what can be observed about the brain would be the clue that solves the puzzle of periodicity. Just such a regularity exists, and there is intriguing and tantalizing evidence that it is crucial. This regularity is alpha rhythm, a brain wave of definable and predictable characteristics which can even be voluntarily controlled, but whose essential nature has still eluded understanding. In recording the electroencephalogram (EEG) from electrodes on the surface of the scalp, alpha rhythm is a 10-cycle-per-second wave (it may vary from 7 to 13 cycles per second in different subjects), most easily found in the occipital area (the part of the scalp just over the visual cortex). Most people's alpha rhythm is either enhanced or caused to appear by closing the eyes, and, for some, by elevating the eyes (Mulholland & Evans, 1966), and is conversely attenuated or entirely stopped by opening the eyes and by concentrating visual attention. Some people almost never show alpha rhythm under any condition while others almost never fail to show it under any condition. Thus people naturally group along a continuum according to the amount of alpha rhythm they show and the conditions under which they show it. Although early efforts to define types of people with much or little alpha rhythm have not been fruitful, it now appears that these studies had not tapped the important dimensions of the personality related to alpha rhythm and that new efforts may prove more successful. In general, it seems that the more intense and the more constantly vigilant a person is, the less alpha he has; and that the more relaxed and casual, the more alpha he will have. Especially exciting is the finding that by being provided with an external psychophysiological feedback which enables a person to know when alpha is present in his brain waves a person may be trained to control his production of alpha (Brown, 1970; Gaarder, 1971b; Kamiya, 1969). By using tension, mental concentration, visual attention, and alertness, a subject may readily block or attenuate his alpha rhythm; while by making his mind blank, by "turning off" or not concentrating upon visual perception, and by trying to feel as relaxed and as "good" as possible, alpha rhythm may be enhanced, although this is more difficult to learn. Thus, the state of the mind is somehow very directly connected with the type of brain waves a person has. Once these matters are understood, they may be simpler than anticipated.

The major reason we are interested in alpha rhythm is because of the relationship between alpha rhythm, processing of information by the brain, and eye jumps. The concept of the brain as a discontinuous information processor has to do with ideas that there are moments when it is more receptive and more capable of transmitting information and moments when it is less receptive and less capable of transmitting information. This is in contrast to the idea of the brain being equally receptive to information throughout any period of time. If the concept of discontinuous processing were literally and simply true there ought to be striking experimental evidence of it; so far such evidence has not been found. Instead, what has been found is evidence (Callaway & Yeager, 1960; Kristofferson, 1967; Lindsley, 1952; Pollen et al., 1971) substantially in favor of the idea of discontinuity, but not straightforward and easy to interpret. This evidence has been diffuse enough so that no solid models leading to general predictions of new experimental results have emerged, and there is consequently no scientific consensus about discontinuity. The reviews of Bertelson (1966), Harter (1967), and White (1963) have described the kinds of evidence and the history of the development of this area of evidence, and have summarized the theorizing and model building which has been done. To understand alpha rhythm better, a few of its time relationships may be considered. Of particular interest is the fact that the alpha frequency can be changed in various ways. One way is by changing the subject's state of consciousness through meditation (Gaarder, 1971a). A lowering of frequency is reported in this situation (Kasamatsu & Hirai, 1966). One importance of this finding for our purpose is that it shows alpha rhythm—as a reflection of intrinsic brain timing relationships—to exhibit lability, with the capacity to adaptively speed up or slow down by large amounts. Thus, if one thinks of alpha rhythm as an "internal clock," it is not a clock with a fixed relation to real time, but one that speeds up and slows down as the occasion requires. This puts it within our definition of cyclicity (Sec. 3.1) and accounts further for the difficulties of demonstrating periodicity.

Another reason for the importance of alpha rhythm is its close relationship with some natural behavioral rates. A consideration of such rates as those of key pressing, drumming with drumsticks, rates of processing visual and auditory information, rates of flicker fusion, and so forth make it quite plain that human function can go somewhat faster than once a second before it breaks down. Much evidence shows that about 10 times per second is a significant psychophysiological period. Since this is the middle of the frequency range of alpha rhythm, there is a major coincidence requiring understanding.

These rates may be studied by considering a very simple example: Tap your finger once per second and notice that this is quite easy to do. Then tap it faster and faster and note that there is a point at which you can tap no faster and that your regularity deteriorates if you try. You will find you cannot go faster than 3 to 5 times a second. Doing this simple experiment may help to clarify these concepts and make them more concrete. Another example illustrating these issues has to do with eye movements. Voluminous work on eye movements in reading has shown a maximum rate of eye jumps in speed reading of 4 to 5 jumps a second (Tinker, 1958). However, the maximum rates are rates established over several seconds of sampling and it is striking how much faster the absolute minimum interval is between two individual eye jumps (Gaarder, 1967b). Here it has been shown that the absolute minimum intereye jump interval is about 50 milliseconds, which would represent a rate of 20 jumps per second if such a minimum interval were sustained. Figure 3.1 helps to clarify this by showing a sample of eye movement record in which the very short 50-millisecond intervals are combined with longer intervals so that in practice the overall mean rate of reading eye jumps turns out to be the lower figure of 4 to 5 per second as against the 20-times-per-second maximum hypothetical rate if each eye jump

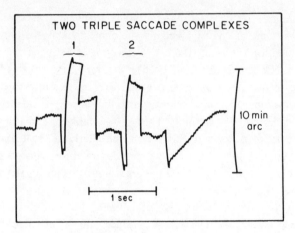

Fig. 3.1. Eye movement record showing minimum inter-jump interval of 50 milliseconds. Two triple eye jump groups (1 and 2) are shown, separated by a single jump between. Within a triple eye jump group the first interval of 50 milliseconds is followed by a second of about 200 milliseconds (From "Some Patterns of Fixation Saccadic Eye Movements" by K. Gaarder, *Psychonomic Science,* 1967, 7, 145–146. Reprinted by permission of the editor.)

had a 50-millisecond interval. These rates also reflect the degree of physiological arousal or alertness which is, of course, related to the speed of information processing and performance. Thus, Gaarder (1967b) has shown a correlation between arousal level and frequency of eye jumps and Hebbard and Fischer (1966) have shown a striking increase of eye jump frequency from about 1 per second in normal states to over 4 per second in the hyperaroused state produced by psychedelic drugs.

What emerges from these findings is a picture of intermittency and discontinuity with its own irregularity, where it is not strictly and regularly periodic. Further clarification of the lack of strict periodicity will follow in Sec. 3.6 when interjump interval histograms are examined. Here, however, what we are doing is underscoring the two issues of discontinuity and of rhythmic alpha brain waves, so as to relate them to one another. So far we have shown that there is a breakdown of performance in the time domain of alpha rhythm and have given some examples within this domain. The major idea put forward to account for the importance of alpha rhythm is that at a certain part of the alpha cycle the brain is more receptive to receiving information than at others (Callaway & Yeager, 1960; Kristofferson, 1967;

Lindsley, 1952). This is interpreted to mean that there is a gate that is open during part of the cycle or that the system's sensitivity threshold is lower at part of the cycle. The importance of these ideas for us is that we now have reason to examine the relationship between alpha rhythm and eye jumps.

3.4. Quasi-harmonic Relations in Brain Waves

Further clues about intrinsic controlling rhythms can come from the study of quasi-harmonic relations of the different components of brain waves. Harmonic relations are well worked out mathematical properties of near-ideal waves, such as sound waves, where simple relationships exist between two waves. For example, musical scales are such that the note of C is 256 cycles per second in one octave and its harmonic in the next higher octave is exactly twice this, or 512. Since the underlying mechanisms of similar findings in brain waves have not been worked out, such relationships should be considered quasi-harmonic, i.e., exhibiting harmonic properties without the unwarranted assumption being made that the mechanisms of sound wave or mathematical harmonies necessarily operate.

Beta rhythm is part of what is called "low voltage fast activity" in the EEG and is the rhythm normally present when alpha is blocked out by opening the eyes in bright light. Its fequency is between 15 and 30 cycles per second and is usually considered the normal brain activity during alert attention. By means of power spectrum analysis it is possible to plot the relative amounts of the energy of a sample of EEG activity which are in the various frequencies. On the basis of a chain of facts, it may be predicted that the frequency of beta rhythm in a given subject should be twice the frequency of his alpha rhythm. The chain of facts upon which this prediction may be made are: (*a*) The minimum interjump interval between eye jumps is 50 milliseconds, which is exactly half of an alpha interval (Gaarder, 1967b). (*b*) When eye jumps are related to the sinusoidal quadrant of alpha waves (see Sec. 4.7), the next highest frequency of eye jumps is often found to be in the quadrant opposite the quadrant with the highest frequency, which again suggests a 50-millisecond interval (Gaarder et al., 1966a). (*c*) A model of a discontinuous, time-shared processor would move in incremented steps (see Sec. 7.5) related to the intrinsic clock. EEG studies of a karate expert executing a movement have shown a frequency of 40 cycles per second (L. Fehmi, personal communication, 1970) while power spectrum studies of expert meditators have shown a peak at the same frequency (E. E. Green, personal communication, 1972). This meets the criterion of a "second harmonic," four times the fundamental frequency. Sokolov (1963) has also described quasi-harmonic frequencies during photic driving, where a 9-cycle-per-second flickering stimulus produced power spectrum peaks at 9, 18, and 27 cycles per second. It is further worth noting that the empirical definitions of the midpoints of the classified brain waves forms a quasi-harmonic series: delta—2½ cycles per second; theta—5 cycles per second; alpha—10 cycles per second; beta—20 cycles per second, and gamma—40 cycles per second.

Quasi-harmonic relations between alpha and beta frequencies are indeed found, as predicted, in many subjects (Gaarder & Speck, 1967). When power spectra of these individuals are examined, the beta peak is exactly twice the frequency of the alpha peak.

The significance to be attached to the fact that brain rhythms exhibit these quasi-harmonic relations is mainly that it lends strength to the idea of cortical periodicity with the interesting addition that periods may occur not only in a basic unit (alpha) but in units one-half and one-fourth the time period of the basic unit. This is important to the idea of unique psychophysiological states with their own particular modes of information processing (Secs. 7.5, 8.2, & 8.3). It also is consistent with an idea of units which may be structured in chains with various multiples (Chaps. 7 & 8). In other words, in one state or at one time the basic unit might be the 50-millisecond beta unit and in another state or at another time it might be the 100-millisecond alpha unit or a 25-millisecond gamma unit. The picture emerging is that not only does the hypothetical "internal clock" show variations based on the speeding and slowing up of alpha rhythm, but that variations may also be anticipated which are related to the quasi-harmonic qualities of the nervous system.

3.5. Periodicity in Eye Jumps

At the simplest level, if eye jumps reflected a periodicity of the brain, it would be expected that examination of the intervals between the eye jumps might reveal the periodicity. A good way of testing this possibility is to construct interjump interval histograms. The way to do this is to take a long segment of eye movement record from a subject and measure all of the intervals between eye jumps. When this is done, one has a series of numbers, each of which represents the time between two eye jumps. These times are then plotted in histogram form, which is a type of graph where the horizontal axis represents the quantity being measured and units on the vertical axis represent the number of events falling in a particular category of the horizontal axis. Thus, time is the horizontal axis of the graph, and it is

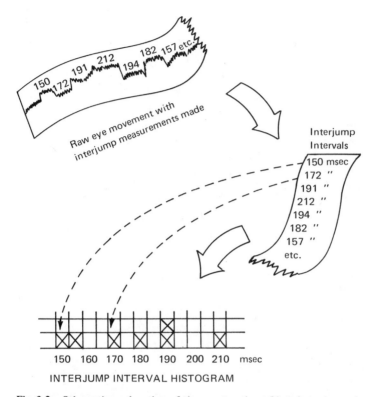

Fig. 3.2. Schematic explanation of the construction of interjump interval histograms. Interjump intervals are measured on the raw record, listed, and then recorded as discrete events on the histogram.

divided into units which would allow a periodicity of 10 or 20 times per second to be detected while the vertical axis measures the number of interjump intervals which fall in a particular time period. Figure 3.2 shows this in more detail.

If a 10-cycle-per-second periodicity were present in eye jumps, it would be expected that the number of jumps occurring at 0.1-second (100-millisecond) intervals would be greater than those occurring at other intervals. Although this is often the case, as in Fig. 3.3, other subject's histograms do not show this relationship. Although many histograms show this periodicity, numerous attempts to detect periodicity in histograms not showing it (by compensating for the various conceivable factors, such as the possibility that basic periods slowly fluctuated over time, and by using various techniques to emphasize periodicity, such as curve smoothing), have been unsuccessful.

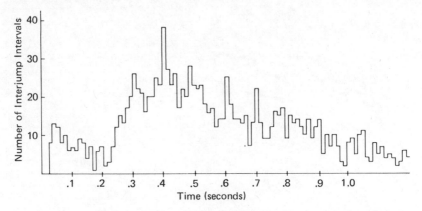

Fig. 3.3. Interjump interval histogram. Note the peaks at or near 0.3, 0.4, 0.5, 0.6, and 0.7 sec.

Various explanations can be offered as to why periodicity is not uniformly detected. Much of the reasoning (Secs. 3.1 & 3.3) points toward cyclicity having its own variance, which is great enough over an interjump interval of several cycles to wash out the signs of the periodicity. This possibility is strengthened by the necessity of a biological rhythm to have built-in variation to prevent the system from fortuitously being thrown into oscillation by external stimulation exactly in time with the intrinsic periodicity. A concrete example may make it clear how variation of the cycle would make demonstration of periodicity difficult. If we assume a basic intrinsic cycle of 100 milliseconds and assume a variability in this cycle of ±10 milliseconds, then an interjump interval of 500 milliseconds, representing an interjump interval of five basic intrinsic cycles of 100 milliseconds, might have a variability of ±50 milliseconds (from 450 to 550 milliseconds). This variability could easily wash out evidence of periodicity in the histogram.

A further source of variability to be noted is that as the eye jumps about, various factors affect the rate at which the new information from a new fixation reaches the brain, which would affect when a new cycle begins. One of the most important of these factors is the intensity of illumination of the new fixation relative to the intensity of illumination of the old fixation. Thus, if someone sits in a dimly lit room on a sunny day and alternately looks out the window and into the interior of the room, the alternate fixation on a brightly illuminated and a dimly illuminated visual world will result in alternate rapid and slower conduction times for messages from the retina to the brain (see Scott & Williams, 1959). There are complex interactions between the time it takes for an eye jump to occur, which is closely related to the size of the eye jump (Zuber, Stark, & Cook, 1965), and the relative amounts of change of luminous flux (J. C. Armington, personal communication, 1972) and the direction of the change (on versus off) (Gaarder, 1968) which may be enough to account for the failure to find periodicity in intersaccadic intervals.

From the standpoint of technique and methods, the universal demonstration of periodicity in interjump intervals will require taking the variability of individual cycles into account. On the other hand, if cyclicity rather than periodicity is acceptable, quite a bit has already been shown.

3.6. Eye Jumps and Alpha

Crucial observations relating alpha rhythm and eye jumps may be made by comparing simultaneously collected records of eye jumps and brain waves, either through tabulation from the raw record or through the use of the computer of averaged transients.

Figure 3.4 is a suitable place to make such observations, which is simply to note that when occipital evoked responses are triggered by the jumps of the eye, the alphalike activity recorded maintains the same phase relationship from sample to sample (Gaarder et al., 1966b). (Phase relation refers to the relative positions of peaks and troughs over time from sample to sample. The concept is derived from trigonometry and elementary wave mathematics by drawing analogy between an alpha wave and a mathematical sine wave. Two sine waves would be said to be "in phase" if their peaks and troughs match each other. Two waves are said to be 180° out of phase with one another if the peaks exactly match troughs and vice versa. The reason for this designation is that a single whole sine wave is defined as covering 360°, so that a half-wave difference is 180°. Waves may be out of phase in varying amounts and this difference is termed "phase lag" [see Sec. 1.6 on time delays]). The fact that alpha rhythm maintains the same phase relation from one sample of eye jump triggered brain activity to another means that there is a relationship between the timing of the phase of alpha rhythm and the timing of eye jumps.

Although the relationship is evident from the simple examination of Fig. 3.4, this is not the only way it may be demonstrated. Another method is to use a simple counting technique to tabulate in which quadrant of alpha each eye jump occurred when evoked responses to eye jumps are recorded under very low illumination (Gaarder et al., 1966b). This method shows a clear

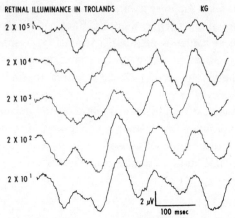

RETINAL ILLUMINANCE IN TROLANDS   KG

2 X 10⁵

2 X 10⁴

2 X 10³

2 X 10²

2 X 10¹

2 μV
100 msec

Fig. 3.4. Phase locking of alpha activity in eye
jump linked evoked responses recorded at different stimulus illuminances. Inion electrode positive downward. (From "The Relation of the
Phase-locked Saccade-linked Component of Alpha
Rhythm to Change of Stimulus Illuminances" by
K. Gaarder, A. Alterman, and W. Kropfl, *Psychonomic Science,* 1966, **5,** 445–446. Reprinted
by permission of the editor.)

tendency for eye jumps to occur in a particular quadrant. A different method
is to compare a large number of samples of eye jump linked brain activity
collected with the CAT. When this is done, subjects show a phase-locked
relationship of their alpha activity (Gaarder, Alterman, & Kropfl, 1966a).

From these studies one may conclude that the occurrence of eye jumps is
definitely related to the particular phase of alpha rhythm. Rather than having
demonstrated periodicity in eye jumps, we have identified their cyclical
nature and their linkage to a rhythm (alpha) which itself lacks the degree of
periodicity to reciprocally result in periodicity in eye jumps.

An important technical point to be made is that so far eye jumps represent
the only available brain output which gives us a synchronizing signal to relate
to the intrinsic rhythms of the brain. Advantage of this is taken in the
experiments demonstrating a relation between eye jumps and alpha just
discussed. Later (Chap. 7) this synchronizing signal will be used to examine
auditory-visual interaction.

3.7. Recapitulation

We can now recapitulate what this chapter has explored. First have been
the issues of periodicity and discontinuity of information input and

processing by the brain. These concepts have been shown to be related to the more general concept of cyclicity and the rhythmicity of brain waves. Cyclicity and discontinuity have then been tied to eye jumps, which were earlier shown to represent a discontinuous process. Thus we have three areas showing overlap—the concept of discontinuity in brain processing, the cyclical nature of brain recordings themselves, and the cyclical discontinuity of function of eye jumps.

Each of the first three chapters has contributed a central idea for our brain model building—the idea of feedback, the idea of discontinuity in eye jumps, and the idea of intrinsic discontinuity in the brain. The next chapter will put these elements together in a model of visual information processing.

4
FURTHER CLARIFICATION OF
THE ROLE OF EYE JUMPS

4.1. Introduction

In this chapter we will sketch out those aspects of the discontinuous feedback model of vision related to the mechanics of eye jumps. This will be done by further elaboration of the concept of discontinuity and by using photographic simulations to demonstrate concretely what occurs on the retina during eye jumps. From this we will have a fairly complete model which later chapters will relate to the overall phenomenon of visual perception.

4.2. Computer Analogies

The simplest way to understand the model and its derivation is by use of some analogies to computing machines which we have already considered (Secs. 2.3 & 3.2). A crucial fact about a given computer is whether it is digital or analog. The word "digital," derived from the Latin word for finger or toe, reflects the fact that just as the fingers represent distinct units (up to ten), so likewise does the digital computer operate upon distinct numerical units rather than along a continuum of an infinite number of steps. On the other hand, the analog computer operates on a continuum and not in discrete units. Part of the reason for using the word analog is the fact that early analog computers literally set up mechanical analogies to the problems they were solving. Not only does the distinction between discontinuous digital and

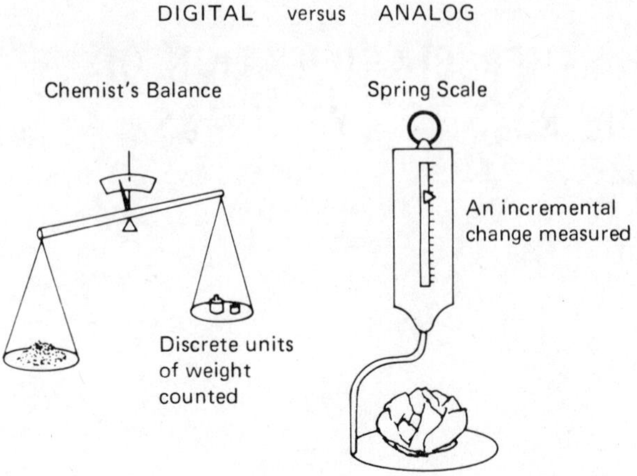

DIGITAL   versus   ANALOG

Chemist's Balance   Spring Scale

An incremental
change measured

Discrete units
of weight
counted

Fig. 4.1.   Examples of the difference between a discrete digital
versus a continuous analog measuring system.

continuous analog affect the units of measurement, as will be discussed now, but it also affects the relationship of time to the units of measurement and to the function of the system of one type or the other. A very simple example of the distinction between a digital and an analog system is the distinction between a simple chemist's balance using a set of discrete weights and an iceman's spring scale (Fig. 4.1). On the chemist's balance, the quantity to be weighed is put on one pan and counterbalanced with discrete unitary weights on the other pan. Since the weights only go down to a certain size, there is a minimum unit of weight below which the chemist cannot measure, determined by the set of weights he has to use. On the other hand, the spring scale measures units along a continuous, unbroken scale, and every increment of weight will be represented along its scale. Other examples of discrete digital devices are such counters as mechanical adding machines and the escapement mechanism of a pendulum clock which can only advance abruptly when the pendulum's swing releases the escapement wheel. Other examples of analog devices are scales such as a ruler or slide rule or the face of a clock where any incremental measurement can hypothetically be made. Digital devices operate by *counting* discrete units; analog devices operate by *measuring* along a continuous scale.

The digital and analog concepts fit naturally to computers, where there are two distinct types, each with its own characteristics. The digital computer always operates upon discrete units in some way, so that any quantity it handles must have a distinct numerical representation in terms of some sort of counting units. The analog computer, on the other hand, only deals in measuring a place along a continuum. Digital computers are built around memory storage spaces, where discrete numbers can be exactly stored, and manipulated as chosen, whereas analog computers are built around continuously processing operational units that do not store discrete quantities exactly, but which handle the infinite increments between two discrete measures on a scale. The effect this has upon time in relation to each is that the digital computer naturally operates in discrete steps over time, whereas the analog computer naturally operates continuously over every moment of time. In other words, the digital computer operates by jumps: jump-stop-jump-stop-jump-stop, etc.; while the analog moves along continuously in infinite increments, so it is always moving. This is an extremely simplified explanation of the distinction between the two types of computers. The purpose is not the understanding of computers per se, for which one might better refer to standard elementary texts (Navweps OP3000, 1963; Westwater, 1962). Rather, I wish to make the distinctions between discrete discontinuous digital systems and continuous infinitely incremented analog systems as concrete and lucid as possible through examples.

Although these distinctions have long been recognized by the mathematician, it is only through the recent widespread use of computers that the distinctions have had the understanding they now enjoy. Prior to popularization of computers, the distinction was only one of a wide variety of logical discriminations that could be made and in no way especially stood out from the rest. Not much is yet understood about the way in which the concrete availability of a concept enables its use in ways that were not possible while it was merely one of a number of abstractions, nor are the advantages of retaining simplicity in thinking fully appreciated.

4.3. The General Problem of the Distinction between the Continuous and the Discontinuous

When considering a given system—be it mechanical, electrical, or biological—in relation to the concepts of continuity versus discontinuity, one of the questions that arises is whether the concepts are being applied to the system per se or to the observation of the system; i.e., is continuity or discontinuity intrinsic to the system or intrinsic to the observations being made upon the system? For example, in the preceding section (Sec. 4.2), we have implicitly assumed that the concepts of continuity and discontinuity are intrinsic to the analog and digital systems. Although there is doubtlessly great value in doing so, it can also be seen that there is some arbitrariness in the application of the concepts. Thus, in studying a given system, we may either choose a conceptual framework with continuity or discontinuity for our attempted understanding (see also Ashby, 1963, p. 28). For example, if we wish to consider a digital computer as continuous, we merely say that the time course of the machine is a continuous one, and that some of the time the movement is to make no movement, while at certain moments when the machine makes a step, that the movement at that point is to make a jumping movement. Or we may take the converse case of an analog computer and argue that if we break its movements down finely enough we will eventually find that they consist of the discrete movement of individual electrons and that therefore the analog computer is "really" digital. These are examples of how the concepts of continuity and discontinuity can be applied to the system per se to attempt to understand the fundamental intrinsic nature of the system. Other instances show how the concepts may apply to the observations made on the system. Thus, if an observer makes a decision about whether to study weight in certain systems using a pan balance or a spring scale, he makes a decision about using digital or analog observational techniques. Likewise, an observer who makes a choice between using a digital or an analog computer to study his problem makes the same choice. What this demonstrates is a dual nature of the concepts of continuity and discontinuity; they may either be attributes of the conceptual framework used to examine a system, or they may be attributed to the system per se, as "natural" or "intrinsic" to the system. These distincitons are elusive and it is important to keep them clear. Nevertheless, it is quite apparent that the concepts of continuous and discontinuous as attributes of analog and digital computers have great value in helping to understand computers.

This leads naturally to the more important question of whether the distinction between the continuous and the discontinuous can help us to understand biological systems. Especially, we are concerned with the question of whether it is useful to assume continuous or discontinuous properties as being intrinsic to a given system. This is the issue, of course, in our earlier attributing the step function to eye jumps (Sec. 2.3) and in attributing intermittency properties to intrinsic brain rhythms (Chap. 3). Studying these questions is difficult because we first must decide to what extent we have already set up an experimental and conceptual framework which predetermines the answer we can receive to our questions. For example, we might ask whether the idea that the brain is a continuous processor has been implicitly taken for granted until recently. Now it would seem that increasing numbers of investigators studying the problem are considering the brain as intrinsically a discontinuous processor. Much greater richness is added to the already elusive issues when it is considered that the system in which we are interested is also an information processing system (see Chap. 5). This, likewise, is only recently being concretely appreciated.

4.4. Is the Visual System Continuous or Discontinuous?

The answer depends on the perspective of the questioner. First of all, as to the subjective nature of vision, there is an implicit shared assumption that the subjective stream of visual perception is experienced as continuous. This important fact of subjective reality has overwhelmingly obscured for us the possibility that the visual process might be intrinsically discontinuous by nature. To press this argument we can marshal two simple observations to show the discontinuous nature of the visual process. One of these observations is to look at oneself in a mirror and alternately direct the gaze at the pupil of one eye and then the other. Since one does not see the eye jump when the gaze shifts, obviously the experienced continuity of vision during the eye jump is illusory in some sense. The other observation is of the facts of motion picture perception. Although what is objectively present is 16 still frames per second, what we perceive is a *continuously* moving picture.

The factor of subjective continuity of perception, when combined with the conceptualization of visual processes in terms of energy dynamics rather than information dynamics (Sec. 5.2) has made it impossible for us to consider until recently the full implications of the idea that the visual process might be discontinuous in nature.

4.5. The Eye Jump as the Step Function Imposing Discontinuity upon the Visual System

In the preceding sections we have been building a foundation for considering the jump of the eye as a crucial factor in the process of vision. By showing that an eye jump is a step function, we have shown how it meets the criterion for the kind of event marking the steps taken by a discontinuous processing system. This is the major thesis of this book: *The visual system is a discontinuous processing system where the discontinuities are usually marked by the occurrence of jumping eye movements.* This is also the central fact of the model of visual perception we are constructing. The next section will show diagrams and photographic simulations to illustrate this fact.

4.6. Photographs and Diagrams Simulating the
Retinal Image Edge Templates Generated by
Eye Jumps—The Case during Visual Fixation

In order to understand what happens in the eye during eye jumps it is convenient to use simulations which can be constructed by using simple illustrative diagrams, photographs, and the combination of the two. These will show what we must assume to be the case from simple geometry and it can quite readily be seen that we are dealing with rather concrete physical realities which must be accounted for in one way or another. These simulations have a simple logical impact that must either be explained as done here, or explained in some other way, which has not yet been done.

When we recall again, as we had shown in Sec. 2.3, that the eye jump meets the criterion of a step function, we may then think in terms of the step function as being preceded and followed by two specific states, which we can consider the "before" and "after" states and designate as t_1 and t_2 arbitrarily. It is worth picturing this in an idealized way (Fig. 4.2) with a simulation of an eye jump. It is also worth reiterating the well-known biological axiom that receptor systems respond mainly to *changes* and to note that the eye jump step function represents an abrupt, sudden, incremental change.

With a clear view in mind of our concern, we may now shift our attention to the retina of the eye and ask what happens there because of the eye jump. This can most simply be visualized with a diagram showing an arbitrary segment of the image of an edge on the retina (Fig. 4.3, Part I). The line

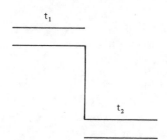

Fig. 4.2. Idealized picture of an eye jump as a discrete step function. t_1 is the time before the eye jump, t_2 is the time after.

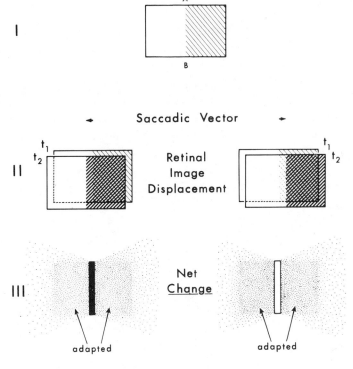

Fig. 4.3. Diagrammatic representation of a segment of retinal image edge information generation by eye jumps. Part I represents the retinal image of a small segment of a vertical edge, A–B, separating a light and a dark area. Part II shows the effects of horizontal eye jump vectors to the left and right on the retinal image. t_1 is the retinal image in the instant before the jump and t_2 is the retinal image in the instant after. Part III shows the net change of this segment of the retinal image generated by the jump. (From "Transmission of Edge Information in the Human Visual System" by K. Gaarder, *Nature*, 1966, **212**, 321–323. Reprinted by permission of the editor.)

between A and B represents an arbitrary segment of edge imaged on an arbitrary portion of the retina. The edge separates the light portion to the left and the shaded portion to the right. There are lines drawn around this in the form of a rectangle for pictorial purposes, but these should be ignored except as necessary to avoid confusion. The next part of the figure, Part II, shows what happens as a result of the movement of the eye when an eye jump occurs. At the top of Part II are shown two arbitrary eye jumps, designated as saccadic vectors (vector is a mathematical term which can be visualized as an arrow where both the length of the arrow and the direction it points have meaning). One eye jump is to the left and the other is to the right. Below each of these is shown the retinal image displacement that accompanies these eye jumps. On the left-hand side is shown what happens when the edge is shifted to the left and on the right-hand side is shown what happens when the edge is shifted to the right. In both cases t_1 is the retinal image before the shift takes place and t_2 is the retinal image after the shift takes place. It is easy to see that there are two classes of before and after conditions on the retinal areas we are considering. (*a*) There are areas in which *no change* takes place; i.e., they are either light before and light afterwards (on the left-hand sides of the retinal area) or they are dark before and dark afterwards (on the right-hand side of the retinal area). (*b*) There are areas in which a *change* takes place—from light to dark or dark to light—as a result of the shift of the retinal image. Part III of the figure shows these last areas of the retina, where a change took place.

The figure can intuitively be seen to illustrate a valid fact. However, it is simplified and leaves out of account such issues as whether the saccadic vector and the retinal image displacements represent the movement of the eye relative to the physical image or vice versa. Clarification of this in no way invalidates the major point of the diagram, however, and is not immediately relevant to our further pursuits.

What has been shown is that small jumps of the eye result in the displacement of edges of the retinal image, wherein the nature of the change produced at the edge is related both to the nature of the edge (i.e., what is on either side of the edge—light versus dark, or red versus green, or plaid versus plain, etc.) and to the direction and size of the eye jump.

So far we have simulated only a single short idealized segment of retinal image edge that does not convey very well what happens over a larger area of the retina with more complex relationships. The purpose of the next figure (Fig. 4.4) is to show this. It is a composite photograph derived from photographing pictures of very simple objects. The same point can be illustrated by photographs or drawings using several different techniques which are illustrated elsewhere (Gaarder, 1968, 1970). It is essential to use very simple objects in the scenes, or the scene quickly becomes too complex to grasp. Thus, the particular simple objects shown were chosen after considerable experimentation. The top two sections of the figure show a "positive" and a "negative" print of the same picture (A is the familiar photograph which we all know, and B is the photographic negative of the same scene). In order to produce the rest of the figure, these two photographs on transparent film are superimposed upon one another and developed onto photographic paper. If the two are placed together with one on top of the other in such a way that every detail corresponds exactly, there would be nothing to see since lights and darks of exactly opposite shades would exactly cancel each other out. This follows a law of photographic technology—that if positive and negative transparencies of the same scene are projected or printed exactly in register (a technical term meaning that all the features match) the result is ideally a uniform shade over the entire area. However, if the positive and the negative transparencies are placed one on the other with a slight displacement (slightly out of register), then patterns of light and dark edges are generated as shown in parts C to H of Fig. 4.4. This is illustrating exactly the same thing as shown in Fig. 4.3, except that a great deal more is shown. It is possible to visualize entire complex figures with this method. It is also possible to see shades instead of just one light and one dark tone and it is possible to see the effect of vectors of different sizes and directions resulting in patterns of edges with different characteristics. In addition, if actual photographs of objects are used for the simulation, it is possible to see interesting texture effects that unfortunately do not reproduce well on printing plates, but that may be relevant to future theories of texture perception.

One important feature of these figures is that a unique set of edges with its own particular combination of lights and darks is produced by each particular eye jump vector. Saying the edges are "unique" means that the set of edges is different if the direction or size of the eye jump is different. For example, Parts E and F in Fig. 4.4 are vectors of almost the exact opposite direction from one another. There it can be seen that each set of edges is almost the exact opposite of the other—where there is a light edge in one there is a dark edge in the other and vice versa. Likewise, these are different than the sets of edges in another vector, such as H. We have here used the terms "unique" and "set" as they are used in set theory (elementary descriptions of set theory may be found in many textbooks, such as Arbib, 1964; Lipshutz, 1964). It is important to note that the sets of edges are unique to the eye jump vector, since the eye jump vector is centrally controlled feedback which, therefore, may select the particular set of edges optimal to the perceptual task at hand. In other words, the particular set of edges transmitted is centrally controlled because the eye jump vector is centrally controlled. These sets of edges may be termed "templates," since this is the term used for a pattern that matches the edges of an object to be reproduced.

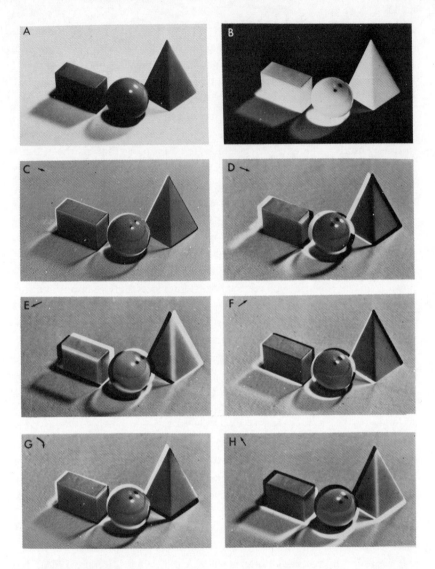

Fig. 4.4. Simulation of retinal image edge information generation by eye jumps. Photo A is a photograph of a simple visual scene. Photo B is the negative of the same scene. When films of A and B are superimposed upon one another with slight displacements, and photographic prints are made, Photos C through H result. This is analogous to what happens on the retinal image when a fixation eye jump takes place. All areas within boundaries which are not crossed "adapt" and are represented by gray. Any border at which light moves to where dark was is represented by a light band, whereas any border at which dark moves to where light was is represented by a dark band. It can be seen that

The main reason these photographic simulations are of interest is that the lights and darks of the edges simulate the momentary lightening and darkening of portions of the retina that takes place when an eye jump occurs; whereas the grays signify areas where no change took place. The light edges obviously fire "on" receptor units on the retina, while the dark edges fire "off" receptor units on the retina. Likewise, in these particular photos where a great deal of edge is present, the specific receptor units fired would certainly be edge detector units that would give information about the directional orientation of the edges from which they were derived. Finally, since the interiors of objects away from the edges are not changed and since the background away from the edge boundaries is not changed, this means that there would be vast areas—the majority of the retina in these photo simulations—where the retinal stimulation would not change and no step function firing would take place. (We are here speaking only of this particular photo.) It is easy to see that each particular visual environment presents its own combination of areas that change and areas that do not change during fixation eye jumps. For example, narrow stripes or concentric rings of circles could present patterns on the retina where almost the entire retina changed. (See Armington et al., 1967, and Harter, Seiple, and Salmon, 1973, for examples of this.)

---

each different vector gives a unique set of edges and that opposite vectors (Photos E and F) give opposite edges.

In order to achieve photographic reproducibility, the vectors have been made larger than might be expected. The arrows near the letter show the approximate direction of movement but do not represent the length of movement accurately. At 15 inches one degree is approximately one-quarter inch. A typical fixation eye jump might result in 1/32 or 1/64 of an inch displacement of a scene viewed at that distance. Therefore, Photo C is most representative of actual magnitudes to be expected. Photos C and D show two vectors of the same direction but different magnitude. This demonstrates the lesser contribution of vector magnitude to the uniqueness of the set of edges. Photo G shows a vector with a torsional component. The right edge of the pyramid therefore shows dark on its upper part and light on its lower.

If the positive and negative films were of exactly the opposite shade at all points, and the areas within boundaries had no texture, a uniform gray should result, but the photographer is unable to achieve this, so that the grays vary in intensity. Although Photos A and B show little texture in the background, it is interesting to note the variety of background textures shown in C through H. (From "Transmission of Edge Information in the Human Visual System" by K. Gaarder, *Nature*, 1966, **212**, 321-323. Reprinted by permission of the editor.)

4.7. Retinal Image Edge Templates Generated by Drifts during Fixation

It will be recalled from Sec. 1.18 that even during eye fixation there continues to be movement in the form of slow drifts and a more rapid tremor. Since the magnitude of the drifts is on the same order of size as the fixation eye jumps, it can be realized upon reflection that the same sort of edge information templates are generated by drift during fixation as are generated by the small eye jumps themselves. There is this important difference: Whereas the edge information templates generated by eye jumps are produced by a sudden displacement along a single vector within a time of 10 to 20 milliseconds, the templates generated by drift occur more slowly over times of from 20 to 1,000 milliseconds and have a shifting vector. This can be recognized as meaning that there would be different retinal and central mechanisms of processing because of the different nature of the temporal stimulation received by the retinal receptors. Earlier work (see review by Alpern, 1972) has suggested that drift is more important than tremor in preventing the disappearance of a stabilized retinal image. In Chap. 6 we will consider the relative places of templates generated by fixation eye jumps and by drifts. For the moment our purpose is merely to observe the fact of these two types of edge templates existing.

Since eye jumps and drifts are of a size of about 5 minutes of arc, this means that these movement may traverse as many as 15 cone receptors. On the other hand, the fine tremor, of about 20 to 30 seconds of arc will traverse about 1 to 1.5 receptors (Alpern, 1972). Whether this produces an effect or not remains to be established by further investigation.

4.8. Photographs and Diagrams Simulating the Retinal Image Templates Generated by Gross Eye Jumps—The Case during Natural Viewing with Large Eye Movements

Everything stated in the preceding section concerning edge information template generation during visual fixation can be appropriately translated to cover the situation during the more usual visual act of letting the eyes jump about a visual environment. (You will recall from Sec. 1.16 that the two cases—of visual fixation and of jumping the eyes about a visual environment—along with the visual tracking of a moving object, effectively cover the most overwhelmingly important possible visual situations.)

Simple observation shows that by far the most common thing for the eyes to do is to jump about with fairly large jumps in the act of perceiving a particular visual environment. Again, recall that to move about in a visual environment, the eye always jumps from one place to another—our discontinuous step function. The eye almost never slowly slides over a scene. It is a worthwhile experiment to try to slowly slide your eyes across a room or across a landscape. Even if you achieved a feeling of success in doing so, you would find if your eye movements were recorded or observed that they were not smooth but were in fact a series of jumps. Although this argument is crucial to the model we are building, we must also keep open to the possibilities of important roles for the exceptions. For example, there are observations by Steinman, Cunitz, and Timberlake (1967) that a subject can on command "hold" his eyes without any eye jumps for periods. Their experiments are now being extended with more sophisticated awareness of the kinds of subjective differences in perception that might result from no eye movements. Also, the growing interest in states of consciousness (Fischer, 1971; Gaarder, 1971a; Tart, 1969) should alert us to the likelihood of different perceptual modes related to different kinds of eye movements.

Figure 4.2, showing a fixation eye movement, would also convey an adequate representation of a gross eye movement by merely changing the vertical scale of the size of the eye movement. Again, the important thing is the fact this is a discontinuous step function. Therefore, each eye jump presents us with a "before" (t_1) and "after" (t_2) situation. Since these facts have been observable throughout history by simply watching another person's eyes as they look about, there must be important reasons why these conclusions were elusive. The subjective continuity of perception (Sec. 4.4) must be one such reason, while the lack of a concrete conceptualization of discontinuous processes (Sec. 4.3) may be another. Using the same reasoning as in Sec. 4.6, we may ask what is happening to the retinal image during viewing of a scene and we may simulate the answer. Figure 4.5 shows a simple scene whose viewing we may consider in Fig. 4.6. Let us imagine that the scene will be projected on a screen for 2 seconds and that an eye is looking at

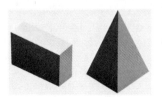

Fig. 4.5. A simple scene to be viewed with simulated gross eye jumps in Fig. 4.6.

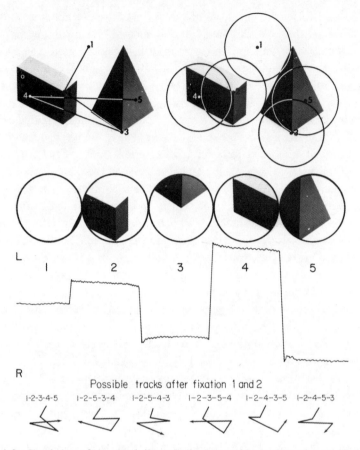

Fig. 4.6. Simulation of the visual discontinuity imposed by gross eye jumps. Upper left is a visual scene with five superimposed spots connected by lines to simulate five fixation points and the track between them. One may assume that the scene is suddenly lit tachistoscopically while the viewer's gaze is at Fixation 1. He then goes to Fixation 2, followed by Fixation 3. These are maximally informative parts of the scene. Having covered these, he goes on to Fixations 4 and 5, ascertaining if he missed anything. This can be considered a "scanning strategy."

The central retinal area covered at each of these five points is schematized on the upper right. The row of circles represents the central retinal area at each of the successive fixations. The purpose of the rows of circles is to convey how the organized percept of a visual scene (upper left) is actually constructed from a discontinuous series of retinal images which we are only capable of integrating as they occur. Underneath the circles is a simulation of the horizontal component of the eye movements making the track along a time base. The horizontal parts of the line represent fixation points while the vertical parts of the line represent eye jumps. L and R designate left and right movements. At the bottom of the figure are all of the possible tracks between the remaining fixation points the screen. The upper left hand side of Fig. 4.6 shows the scene with five connected numbered dots. These five dots simulate five fixations a subject's eye might make in viewing the scene; the five lines signify the eye jumps the subject would make from one fixation to the next. Let us assume that Fixation 1 is where the eye rested before the scene was projected, while the screen was still blank. Because of a latency period before the eye could jump, this would be the first fixation after the scene was projected. Fixations 2 and 3 would be jumps to points of maximal information in the scene. (The information is maximal because the most numbers of edges and surfaces meet at these points.) We know from work by Mackworth and Bruner (1966) and Noton and Stark (1971a, 1971b) that in viewing a scene the eye tends to fixate on points of maximum information. In such a simple scene there isn't much to see, however, so we have arbitrarily decided to have our hypothetical eye go to Fixations 4 and 5, near the periphery of the scene just to make sure nothing has been missed. We now have five fixations separated by large eye jumps, that can be analyzed. Let us now ask how the retina and the brain process this information. As mentioned in Sec. 1.17, the density of retinal receptors and, therefore, the visual acuity, drop off drastically as one moves away from the fovea to the periphery of the retina (Millodot, 1966). If we arbitrarily draw a circle about a fixation point we will arbitrarily define the size of a certain amount of retinal image which could encompass that particular part of the picture within the circle. The purpose of doing this is to show what is around the center of the retina during each of the fixations. Our five fixations will fairly well represent what the eye might have done during the 2 seconds it viewed the scene.

The next part of Fig. 4.6 is a horizontal row of circles. This was made by reproducing the contents of the circles around each of the 5 fixation points in order, as you can see by looking between any circle in the row of circles and the corresponding circle on the upper right. The purpose of this row of circles is to give a concept of the time sequence of events upon the central retina in our hypothetical viewing of the scene of Fig. 4.5. In the preceding section, we saw how fixation eye jumps result in the generation of edge information templates. In this simulation, we can see how it is justifiable to think of each fixation between eye jumps as resulting in the generation of a new package of

---

after Fixations 1 and 2 have occurred. The purpose of this is to show the intrinsic stochastic nature of even a simple scanning strategy. (From *Early Experience and Visual Information Processing in Perceptual and Reading Disorders* edited by F. A. Young and D. B. Lindsley, Washington, D.C.: National Academy of Sciences, 1970.)

information upon the retina. The reason for thinking of it as a package is because of its well defined temporal boundaries, which are brought out by use of a chain of circles across the page simulating the time dimension. The row of circles not only simulates the sequences of events upon the retina but also represents in its essentials how the visual information passes through the lateral geniculate body and the first stage of visual cortical processing. Then, however, because of our much greater subjective comfort with Fig. 4.5 as a whole rather than with the actual breakdown of the scene as the brain processes it, we must assume that at some later stage of the visual process, the chain of Fig. 4.6 is recombined into the whole of Fig. 4.5. (Elsewhere [Gaarder, 1968], the same figure has an additional row of circles under the first. The two rows of circles both show the same sequence, but the second row is modified to attempt two further simulations. The first simulation is the lesser acuity of the peripheral retina. This is achieved by having diffusion of the edges near the rim of the circle. The second simulation is a possible mechanism of comparison of the immediate retinal image with the imme-diately preceding negative afterimage as a means of achieving constancy of the visual world. This is done by superimposing the negative image of the preceding fixation upon any given fixation. Neither of these two points is easily illustrated, so that the second row of circles has not been included in Fig. 4.6.)

The next part of the figure is a simulation of a recording of the horizontal component of the eye jumps shown in two dimensions on the upper left. The L and R designate left and right direction of jump and the numbers refer to the fixation numbers. Those places where the trace is horizontal represent fixation, shown by dots on the upper left; those places where the trace goes nearly vertical represent eye jumps, shown by the connecting lines of the upper left. Since time is the horizontal axis of the recording, it shows better than the upper left how most of the time is spent fixating, with relatively little time consumed by eye jumps.

Finally, the bottom of the figure shows the "possible tracks after Fixations 1 and 2." Here it is assumed that the same fixations are made, but that the sequence of the last three covers all possible combinations of the three as shown above each track. The purpose of this is to demonstrate the extraordinary richness of possibilities of the visual act. We have considered only five possible fixation points out of the infinite number within any scene. By simply rearranging their order we have reintroduced much more complexity of processing sequences. This illustrates how there is an intrinsic stochastic time series involved in the visual process.

One of the most important and typical activities in which gross eye movements are used is reading (Sec. 1.17), simulated in Fig. 4.7. Part I is a small sample of reading text for use in our simulation. Part II shows a set of hypothetical fixations upon the text that a reader might make while reading that text. Here again, the dots represent the fixation points which the fovea of the eye makes. However, as a matter of convenience, curved arrows are used to show the jumps rather than the straight arrows of the preceding figure. The next part of the figure, Part III, shows circles that represent

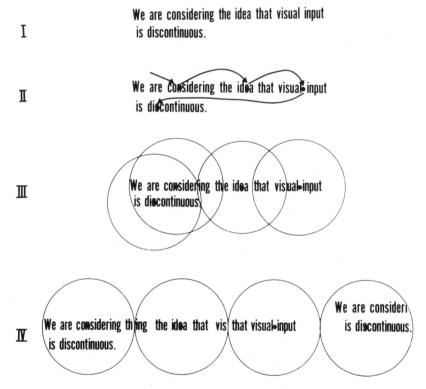

Fig. 4.7. Simulation of the effect of eye jumps during reading. (I) A short sample of text. (II) Simulation of a set of four eye fixations (dots) and the intervening eye jump tracks (arrows) during reading of the text. (III) Simulation of arbitrary central retinal areas about each fixation. (IV) Simulation of the time sequence of presentation to the brain of the chain of four successive central retinal views. Note "overlap" or repetition of certain words during succesive fixations. (From *Early Experience and Visual Information Processing in Perceptual and Reading Disorders* edited by F. A. Young and D. B. Lindsley, Washington, D.C.: National Academy of Sciences, 1970.)

arbitrary central retinal areas around each of the fixations. Part IV shows the chain of circles that represents the time series of events occurring with each successive fixation. It is somewhat easier here to conceptualize how the eye is able to coordinate with the brain the incoherent contents of these four circles automatically into the smooth-flowing sentence of Part I. There is certainly much left to study in attempting to understand this process. However, it is inescapable that an increase in understanding will begin by the tangible recognition of the fact that the reading process shares in common with other visual processes the packaging of information into units by the mechanism of jumping the eye (Wells & Schmaustwein, 1968).

4.9. Recapitulation

To recapitulate what we have learned from our simulations, we can list the following points:

1. We have shown concretely how we may generalize between the gross eye movement of ordinary viewing, the gross eye movements of reading, and the small jumps of visual fixation to cover the most common ways of using the eyes.

2. We have seen how the result of each eye jump is a unique product of the eye jump—of its vector and of where it puts the eye.

3. We have a concrete basis for combining the idea of unique eye jumps with the idea of feedback, since the eye jumps are centrally controlled.

4. We have seen how the step function's discontinuous, incremental effect upon the visual process is to result in the packaging of information.

Before it is possible for us to synthesize adequately what we now know into a more complete model of vision it will be necessary for us to go afield once more to examine in closer detail the problem of information. In Chap. 5 we will examine analogies between the information-carrying capacities of a language and the information-carrying capacities of the visual system, and from that be in a much stronger position to construct a solid model of vision in Chap. 6.

5
THE ORGANIZATION
OF INFORMATION IN
A MODEL OF VISION

5.1. Introduction

To this point, we have built a model of the visual process that relies upon known properties of the visual system, upon predictive experiments, and upon generalizations concerning feedback systems. Now we will add to our consideration a broader view of information theory and will introduce the concept of hierarchy as an essential element in a model of visual information processing. From this we will be able to understand the importance of organization of information.

5.2. The Emergence of the Concept of Information

The concept of information and its detailed elaboration began to be widely known among scientists during World War II as Shannon (1948), Wiener (1948), and others laid out fundamental laws. Just as the concept of feedback had profound impact upon thinking in the biological sciences, so, likewise, has there been far-reaching change in accommodation to the concept of information. Although many of the changes resulting from the use of the concept of feedback have had to do with the demonstration of specific feedback mechanisms, the same is not quite the case with the concept of information. It has been found difficult to use the concepts of information theory to demonstrate concrete manifestations of information in biological systems. Instead, there has been a reorientation of thinking in which information and the laws of information are accepted as a frame of reference. Much of the reason for this is because the general laws of information as derived from nonliving systems are even less translatable to living systems than are the general laws of feedback. Thus, there is widespread intuitive recognition of the importance of informational concepts at the same time as there is acknowledgment that the concepts as now known cannot be directly applied.

One way of understanding the impact of the concept of information is to consider the contrast between the energy dynamics of a system and the information dynamics of the same system (see Ashby, 1963, p. 3). Obviously, in order to transmit and operate upon information, energy is required. However, from the informational point of view, the importance of energy is not for its own sake, but merely because some small quantities of energy are always required to process information. Thus, all real information machines use energy, but the nature of the energy sometimes becomes trivial. For instance, one may add two numbers with an abacus, a mechanical calculator, or an electronic computer. In all cases, analogous informational transactions are carried out and the same answer is reached, even though in each case the energy required to carry out the operations is quite different. An example from biology is the energy of nerve spikes versus the information of nerve spikes. Those familiar with neurophysiology know that a large proportion of recent effort in the field has been devoted to study of the energy characteristics of nerve spikes—membrane potentials, transmitter chemicals, synaptic mechanics, etc. However, we still know practically nothing about the informational dynamics of nerve spikes and still find it difficult even to begin to say what sort of a code is being used, for instance. Thus, while there are some hints, such as finding that rate of nerve spikes is a code in some systems (Harmon & Lewis, 1966; Moore, Perkel, & Segundo, 1966), the further details of how information is transmitted are simply unknown. Another example that is well known is the energy of the evoked response versus the information carried by the evoked response (Uttal, 1965). These issues are brought out by studies (Gaarder, 1968) where evoked responses to eye jumps producing "on" and "off" changes are analyzed by tabulation of amplitudes and wave forms. This is a crude attempt to measure the effect of an informational change (an "on" versus an "off") upon the energy output of the system—the evoked response. Even here there is an energy difference in the "on" and the "off" informational change that might be misleadingly felt more important than the information itself. One point of such examples is to show that biologists are experiencing great difficulty with the conceptual problems of adding the consideration of information to our present capacity to consider energy. This is partly a problem of adapting to a recent advance of fundamental knowledge. It is partly a problem of how we design our models and our experiments. And, as the next section (Sec. 5.3) will show, it is partly a problem of the kinds of units we are capable of dealing with.

Another way of understanding the contrast between energy dynamics and informational dynamics is to consider an analogy. Suppose a large computer were discovered that was programmed in an unknown way to work on an unknown problem and two engineers were set to work to deduce what the computer was doing. Assume one of the engineers was a power engineer and the other an information engineer and each was committed primarily to his own discipline. Assume it was possible for them to monitor the operations of the computer at several internal points, such as the power supply, the accumulators, and the registers, and that it was possible to control the inputs. From the outlook of the power engineer, he would be quite happy to be able to vary the quantities of the input, i.e., to control their energy and find corresponding changes in the points he monitored. Thus, if he applied two inputs, one of which was twice as long as the other and found twice the power was taken to handle the longer one, this would be a valid relationship. Or if he put two quantities through a register and it required proportionately more power to the register to process the larger one, he would be satisfied. On the other hand, the information engineer would be unable to stop with this kind of solution. He would require knowledge to be gotten from such experiments, but he would have to translate the knowledge into terms having to do with information and its coding, rather than leaving it in terms of energy. Thus, he would want to know such things as whether a binary code was in use, what the size of the memory storage units might be, or which registers had access to what parts of memory. A great deal of this kind of knowledge would be necessary before he could even begin to guess what program was being used by the computer—what it was up to.

Our two engineers are analogous to two of the branches of visual science. The older branch is concerned with the energy dynamics of the visual system, and in fact many of its workers are also trained in power engineering and use its concept in deriving their major concerns. Only more recently are visual scientists coming to have the outlook of the informational engineer—first, through the concerns of electronic engineering with the dynamics of circuitry; and, more recently, through outright commitment to strictly informational questions.

5.3.   The Issue of Units—in General
and in Relation to Information

It is a truism of modern science that revolutionary advances most often are organized around fundamental changes in our understanding of the appropriate units for studying a phenomenon. For example, as long as chemistry and physics were operating solely with ordinary units of mass, no fundamental jumps beyond alchemy were possible. However, once the atomic table evolved with the concepts of intrinsic units of protons, neutrons, electrons, atoms and molecules, chemistry fell into place around these organizing concepts of intrinsic units. A similar situation exists in the biological sciences where progress will be made when we become able to deduce fundamental units to understand biological phenomena. At this point it appears likely that appropriate biological units will be informational units rather than units of mass or energy, as in other sciences.

In order to understand this further, we will refer briefly to information theory to show how it has resulted in expanding our basic arbitrary units of mass, energy, and time to include arbitrary units of information. (The interested reader can obtain a nonbiological grasp of this area by reading Shannon [1948]; Ashby [1963] and Wiener [1948] provide further background.) Arbitrary nonbiological units of information include the "bit" or binary digit of information and computer sciences; the "set" of set theory; the channel capacity of information theory; the constraints of set theory and information theory; and the entropy of information theory. Some of these arbitrary units are compound units which means they consist of several components. For example, channel capacity is often expressed in bits per minute, compounding units of information (bits) and units of time (minutes). Information theory may be viewed from our perspective as having added a new dimension to science and what we have referred to thus far may be looked upon as representing some of the arbitrary units of information.

We now come to the problem of what would represent fundamental, intrinsic, natural units of information in a biological system. In order to understand this better, we shall make extensive use of an analogy to be developed between (a) the units and the hierarchical structure of formal printed language and (b) the units and hierarchical structure of visual information. (This treatment is similar to one used by Polanyi [1968] to explain boundary conditions.) In making the analogy we shall refer to both printed language and the visual system as being "information-bearing systems." The reason for choosing this particular term is that the word "bearing" is somewhat broader than other terms, allowing both for the case of information transmitting systems and informational systems that merely exist without actual transmission. This helps to avoid bogging down with the distinction between a printed language that for the most part is seen as it merely exists, and the dynamic visual system that is always transmitting.

In this section we have stressed the importance of intrinsic, natural units to fundamental understanding. We have decided that in biological systems such units must be informational. In the next section we will deduce what such units might be by the use of analogies between language and visual information.

5.4.   Units and Hierarchy in Formal Printed Language

We will begin our development of the analogy between language and vision by describing in detail the characteristics of formal pringed language with which we are concerned, such as printed English. "Formal" means we are concerned only with certain aspects of that printed language's obvious structure and not with such important questions as how it might be psychophysiologically translated internally in reading. (In so doing we do not at all imply these are not important questions, but merely that they are not relevant to the line of reasoning being pursued.) The first of the details of formal printed language, *intrinsic units*, has already been referred to in Sec. 5.3. The other major details are *hierarchies of levels* and *chains*. The meanings of these will become clear as we proceed. We will also make use of set theory terminology in order to clarify some of the relationships. (The concept of hierarchy is complex, as can be appreciated by considering some of its usages: to describe similar units carrying out different graded tasks, e.g., an army of officers and soldiers; to describe higher units composed of lower units, e.g., a visual system made of retinal cells, brain cells, lens cells, etc. The theoretical elaboration of hierarchy is a recent matter of concern [Pattee, 1973; Whyte, Wilson, & Wilson, 1969], as the need of the concept in information theory and biology has become more apparent. Here we are not concerned with the topic of hierarchy in general, but mainly with the topic of hierarchy in the structure of information-bearing systems. Thus, much that is central to the general topic of hierarchy does not concern us and much of what we do consider is not well worked out in the general treatment of hierarchy. It is hoped that most of our use of the concept will be clear in our usage.)

Figure 5.1 shows what we will be working with. In formally describing a printed language we begin at the lowest level of the hierarchy (Level I) by

HIERARCHY OF LEVELS OF PRINTED LANGUAGE

LEVEL

I	a set of letters (alphabet)	(a,b,c,d,e,...,x,y,z.)
II	a set of words ("dictionary")	(and,bird, came,doors, top,...etc.)
III	a set of sentences (ruled by grammar)	(Jack rolled the ball.,Don't eat mushrooms...,etc.)
IV	a set of texts (ruled by style)	(all articles,all books, all manuals,etc.)

Fig. 5.1. Illustration of units and hierarchy in a formal printed language.

noticing that we are dealing with a set of printed letters, which can be called an alphabet. The fact it is a set can merely be taken to mean that it is a well defined collection of objects. Thus, the English alphabet is extremely well defined; it is one of the few areas about which there is virtually unanimous agreement that it consists of the well known 26 letters. (We will simplify our treatment of the subject by ignoring such questions as whether to also include spaces and punctuation marks as members of the set or whether to put them in a separate set which together with the set of the alphabet forms subsets of another set.) A further thing to notice about the set of the letters of the alphabet is that the letters are, in a very real way, each discrete, discontinuous, *intrinsic units* of printed language (each letter has a unitary nature and is intrinsic to the natural structure of the language). A final thing to note about them is that their important characteristic is information rather than energy or mass. In other words, the important thing about an alphabetic letter is how much information it carries, which is related to the size of the alphabet it belongs to and its frequency of use. The fact there is weight to the ink used or energy expended by the press to form the letter or by a transmitting system to send the letter is irrelevant to its informational function as are other measures of mass and energy.

We may now move from Level I, the set of letters, to Level II, the set of words. Here we will find that the reason for describing a hierarchy becomes more evident. Each of the moves we will make from level to level will take us from one group of formal characteristics to another, but the same kind of descriptions will apply in each case. Thus, there will be other *intrinsic units* at Level II; another *set* at Level II; and another *size of set* at Level II. The elements of the set will continue to retain their discrete, discontinuous, intrinsic unitary characteristics and will be important for their information-bearing aspects rather than for energy or mass differences.

Level II is a set of words. English words are formed by combining letters in a *chain*. In other words, the elements of Level II, words, are built of chains of the elements of Level I. In the case of formal printed English the set would include all of the words used in the English language, so that the size of the set would be approximately the number of words in the dictionary, and "dictionary" would be an appropriate descriptive term for the set.

In order to acquire a common sense feeling for the concept of set, and in order to have a further feeling for some of the issues raised by our analogy, we can also note that the set of words of the English language is a subset of a much larger set, which is the set of *all* possible combinations of the letters of the alphabet. Here also, one may gain some feeling for the sizes of sets. Remember that the alphabet had 26 letters, i.e., was a set of 26 elements or members. This is a small and easily handled set, but by building these elements of letters into chains to form words, we have a much larger set which has thousands of elements (words). If we were to consider not only the combination of letters into English words, but also the combination of letters into nonwords, we would again be considering a set which is much larger than the last. What we then consider is the set of all combinations of the letters of the alphabet of which the English dictionary is only a subset. This larger set not only includes *and* and *cat* and *ball* from the English dictionary, but also includes such nonsense words as *xft, drqxb,* and *eee.* We may pause a moment to note that if the sizes of the nonsense words are below a definite number of letters, this set would be a *finite* set, because there would be a limit to the number of possible combinations (even though that limit might be difficult to comprehend for the mathematically unsophisticated), whereas if the size of the nonsense words has no limit the set is an *infinite* one, since no matter how large, the set can always be made larger by adding another letter to the nonsense word.

We are also in a position to consider another issue, dealt with by Shannon (1948). This is the concept of constraint. If we count the frequency of occurrence of each of the letters of the alphabet in any text, we will find that the frequency is very high for certain letters, such as e and other vowels and such consonants as s, t, and h, whereas it is very low for such consonants as x, q, and z. This represents constraint upon an idealized situation in which the frequencies of occurrence of all letters in the set would be equal. At the level of words, we can consider the dictionary as a constraint upon the set of all possible letter combinations into words, and within the set of the words in the dictionary we will also find constraint in any given text, with a much greater probability of the word *the* appearing in a text than the word *obelisk*. Constraint causes structure to exist. We could partially define structure as the manifestation of constraint in a given situation. For example, we may consider the structure which makes up the word *cat*. This word is formed by combining the three letters *a, c,* and *t*. These three letters may be combined in six different ways to form three-letter words, however. Thus we have these possible combinations: *cat, cta, act, atc, tac*, and *tca*. Structure reflects the constraint upon all possible combinations of the letters.

Another fact about the set of words which differentiates it from the set of letters has to do with the size of the units (i.e., the size of the elements or members of the set). In the set of letters, each unit (i.e., each letter) is of equal size. In the set of words, each unit is of the size which may or may not be the same as another unit. Thus we have words with two letters, three letters, four letters, etc., and while each word is a unit (from the standpoint of information bearing) or an element or member (from the standpoint of set theory), the units are not all of the same length (from the standpoint of the number of letters they contain). Consideration of this makes the final point about the level of words—that we are here also dealing with discrete, discontinuous *units*. That is, each word is a unit of information in the formal sense, and the unit is discrete and discontinuous and is also intrinsic to the system rather than arbitrary, but units may differ in size.

In summary, Level II of the hierarchy, the level of words, consists of the enormously large *set* of words, that can be called the "dictionary," the elements of which are also discrete, discontinuous, intrinsic units of the information-bearing system, although of variable size. We have also gained a bit of feeling for the concepts of "set" and "constraint" in the process and have hints of the idea of chains.

We next move to Level III of the hierarchy, which is the level of the set of sentences. Just as words are formed of chains of letters, so are sentences formed of chains of words. The set of sentences is all of the possible combinations of the words of the dictionary that follow the rule of grammar. Thus, an appropriate, if somewhat awkward, descriptive term for the set is "ruled by grammar." This includes such sentences as "Jack rolled the ball," and "Don't eat mushrooms," but excludes nonsensical combinations such as "Pitch role flooding," which does not obey rules of grammar. The size of the set is again very large indeed, many orders of magnitude larger than the size of the dictionary. However, if one specifies a maximum number of words in a sentence, the size of the set of sentences is not an infinite number—merely too large for a small army of people to encounter in several lifetimes. The concept of constraint again appears in sentences. Thus, the rules of grammar are constraints upon all possible combinations of words. One example is in constructing sentences, where the rules of grammar constrain the ordering of words. For example, if we start with the set of words, *the, cat, ate, the,* and *mouse* they make a good sentence in their existing order—*The cat ate the mouse.* However, if the words are rearranged, they do not do so well—*ate mouse cat the the,* or *mouse the ate cat the* are considered nonsensical. Constraint is that which excludes these nonsensical possibilities and structure is the result.

The final things to note about the set of sentences is that each sentence is also a unit of information in the same formal sense as each letter and each word, and these units are likewise discrete and discontinuous. Also, as was true of words, these units are not always of equal size—sentences vary in the number of words making them up.

In summary, Level III, the level of sentences, is made up of the set of all possible sentences, and is therefore enormously larger than the dictionary. The set of sentences is defined by the rules of grammar, that act as a force of constraint giving structure to sentences as opposed to all possible combinations of words. The sentence is an information-bearing unit which is discrete and discontinuous.

We move to Level IV more for the sake of illustrating that higher levels exist than for the sake of tangible understanding. We have previously ignored a number of ambiguities and are now ignoring even more. Earlier we arbitrarily excluded punctuation marks and spaces from the set of letters. We ignored the possibility of syllables as an intermediate level of units between letters and words. We also ignored phrases as an intermediate level of units between words and sentences. We are not saying that these intermediate levels are not important. We are merely saying that the particular levels we have chosen illustrate, with the least confusion, the points we wish to make. In going to a level higher than sentences, we are ignoring paragraphs and chapters as possible units by choosing "texts" as a descriptive term for all articles, all books, all manuals, etc., that are complete in themselves. These are ruled by "style" as a descriptive term to help define the limits of the set of texts. The size of this set is enormously larger than the set of sentences and the set is again made of units of greater and lesser size—some articles are one page long while some books are over a thousand pages long. It is also possible to see that there are hierarchical levels above this one also, such as a "life's work" or a "school" of thought or the chain of printed works leading to a particular product. However, the logical problems of dealing with these have expanded enormously and our sanity is best protected by ignoring them.

One final aspect of this hierarchy of sets requires mention. This is the nature of the information that can be handled at each level. At the level of the alphabet the mathematical information theorist is most at home, because he has very tangible measurements he can make upon the 26 letters with respect to the size of the set, the frequency of occurrence in typical texts, etc. (see Shannon, 1948.) At the level of words he is still somewhat at home and has a contribution to make. However, when we reach the level of sentences, there is little to be gotten from him. Part of this has to do with the nature of the information that can be carried at each level. Letters of the alphabet can convey a certain quantity of information, but the information in and of itself is not of relevance to anything other than the alphabet itself. By combining letters into words, a great deal broader scope of information can be dealt with. Thus, while the letter *b* is merely the letter *b*, the word *airplane* has reference to a whole category of things outside of itself. Likewise, the word *airplane* only refers to a class of things while the sentence *Airplane traffic over Kennedy Field is increasing*, conveys an enormous amount no single word could convey. Although there is no simple system for conveying these differences in level of information, we can easily appreciate intuitively that such differences exist. While information theory defines information very precisely at the level of letters and words, when one reaches the level of sentences things become fuzzy and science is not yet of much help in differentiating a poem from a prescription.

5.5. Information-bearing Systems Generalized

From what we have seen of printed English as an information-bearing system, we can raise some questions and provide tentative answers about information-bearing systems in general. Our purpose in doing so is not to study the general issues for their own sake, but to show a suitable basis for utilizing the analogy we will draw to the visual system.

The major question has to do with asking what sorts of information-bearing systems are intrinsically hierarchical. The other questions are more or less derived from this one. From our analysis of formal printed English we saw how that particular system was intrinsically hierarchical. In other words, the organization of that particular information-bearing system was structured into levels of increasing complexity where the units of a higher level are made up of a number of the units of a lower level. These units were intrinsic in the sense that they were themselves the unitary building material of the system at the same time as they had informational representation in their particular form as they stood. In printed English these units are discontinuous at all levels and are formed into chains.

Further strength for our argument about discontinuity would be gained if it were possible for mathematical logicians to resolve whether an information-bearing system which is discontinuous at a lower level is constrained to be discontinuous at all higher levels. Intuitively and by our example it would appear to be so, but it may be possible to study the question logically. The discontinuous alphabet apparently constrains words, sentences, and higher printed units to be discontinuous, and it would be revealing to know if discontinuous nerve spikes likewise constrained all higher nervous informational units to be discontinuous.

When all hierarchical information-bearing systems are considered together, it is not specified how time is related to chains. Thus, considering a printed sentence as it exists on a page, the sentence as a thing in itself exists over time. However, in order to process a long sentence, it is necessary to deal with it in some serial fashion. In other words, few systems, and certainly no living systems (human readers), would take in the whole sentence as an instantaneous whole (entirely parallel processing). Instead, the typical way of processing a sentence is to start at the beginning and move on to the end (serial processing). Thus, when we are not considering the structure of information-bearing systems as things in themselves which exist over time, we must consider some laws of processing which in the case of printed English turn out to be based on some sort of serial processing where units are read-in over time. (We are neglecting here to go into the neurophysiology of reading, in which it would be found that whole words and even short phrases may be processed in parallel as units. However, in this case it could be shown that the original learning process had involved a serial processing of letters, so that before learning had been completed, time had been an important factor.)

The above properties—*of lawful hierarchy of increasing complexity, intrinsic units, discontinuity, chains, and seriality which may be temporal*—are the issues whose generality we wish to study. In order to examine this a bit further we can first attempt a classification of information-bearing systems. Since this is a side issue to our central task of understanding vision, we will not do so exhaustively. However, a tentative classification of information-bearing systems may be made into the living and the nonliving.

The living systems would include man with his visual system, of course, and all other living organisms as well. The nonliving systems would include those that are made by a living system and those that exist by themselves apart from living systems.

A few examples of each of these classes of information-bearing systems will help us orient ourselves. First, as to living systems, man or an ape or an ant are all examples. They are all information bearing in an extreme degree and are all complex and made up of many levels. To be more concrete, we can take the circulatory system of man as another example of a living information-bearing system. There are several finite information-bearing homeostatic mechanisms operative in the circulatory system; an example is the blood pressure regulatory mechanism (thus we have moved down in another type of hierarchy—man to circulatory system to blood pressure regulation). The blood pressure regulating system has receptors, transmitting elements, and effectors which taken together constitute an information-bearing system.

From this sparse description of hierarchy in a living system, it will not be difficult to attribute the property of lawful hierarchy of increasing complexity to living systems from the standpoint of most current scientific philosophies. Once viewed from an informational standpoint, intrinsic units in serial chains can also be seen as the most likely possibility.

In considering nonliving systems, we can leave out of account those systems which are not man made, such as the cosmos, since it is unclear exactly how it is an informational system and its exact relevance to our humble task is obscure. Among manmade systems we can already utilize the extensive analysis of formal printed English as providing an example of the properties we are studying. In contrast we can point to another manmade information-bearing system as not containing the properties we are studying. This is the simple glass lens, wherein the information in light rays is collected and reorganized into a new optical image. Here there is no hierarchical structure—only a one-for-one transformation of geometrical structure. Likewise, there is no increasing complexity since there is no hierarchy. Also, the units of information are not intrinsic to the lens as a system, but instead are intrinsic to the organization of light in the original image and its scatterings. Further, the concepts of discontinuity, chains, and seriality are somewhat meaningless to this system. It is important to recall that the simple lens and its image is one of the primary analogical models of the visual system from which we have derived much of our knowledge, since it helps us to understand why the contrasting hierarchical properties with which we are concerned have received such little consideration until information theory became available.

What our analysis of the general properties of information-bearing systems has now demonstrated is that all systems do not show the properties of hierarchies of increasing complexity, etc. The simple lens is a striking example of an information-bearing system without the properties we are studying. We can also recognize how the analogy to the simple lens has shaped our previous models of the visual system (Gaarder, 1963) and how we are now faced with choosing between the two types of models of information-bearing systems in modeling the visual system.

5.6. The Visual System as
an Information-bearing System

We shall now return to the visual system and apply some of the principles we have extracted from our study of printed language and the derived hypothetical generalizations. We will do this by considering each of the properties with which we concerned ourselves in Secs. 5.4 and 5.5 –hierarchy, intrinsic units, discontinuity, chains, and seriality.

Hierarchy in the visual system is not a thoroughly studied issue. One reason would seem to be the strength of the intuitive analogy between ordinary photographs and visual percepts. In considering a photograph, hierarchy is not an immediately appropriate concept. Certain things in the real world are faithfully reproduced in geometrical relation to one another on a piece of paper. The reproduction of exact structural relationships is an easily understood mechanical matter and ideas about information appear somewhat superfluous, the more so if the informational concept is hierarchy. Therefore, to the extent that the visual system is a camera and the visual percept a photograph (Gaarder, 1963), we are not in need of a concept of hierarchy in the visual system.

Hierarchy in the visual system must have its own experimental and pragmatic base of evidence to support it before it can be accepted and we will now look at this briefly. One such basis would be found in the empirical data concerning the microgenesis of visual percepts (Flavell & Draguns, 1957). According to these observations, very brief tachistoscopically flashed pictures are not well perceived in their entirety. In other words, you can't see it all in a momentary flash. This is interpreted in terms of finite amounts of time being required to build up the complete percept from hierarchically lower units. Another argument in favor of hierarchy has to do with the idea of coding and recoding of visual information at the retinal and lateral geniculate synapses. Such a visual phenomenon as lateral inhibition in receptor units would in one sense represent a coding of information, which is a different process than the simple straightforward one-for-one transformation of silver salt granules on a photographic plate. An elaboration of this idea which also favors hierarchy is the near certainty that the visual system transmits much more information about *edges* where changes take place, than it transmits about central areas away from edges where no change takes place (see Fig. 4.4, for example). Such a process also shows how the simple one-for-one transformation of the photograph is not adequate.

Another reason for favoring a concept of hierarchy can be seen by studying the figures which simulate gross eye movements.

If you look at Fig. 4.5, you will see an integrated whole, which, however, the parts of Fig. 4.6 explain to be the result of putting together separate pieces that degenerate in acuity away from their central foveal areas. Likewise, in the process of reading, Fig. 4.7 shows how a continuous reading of a text comes from the unequal jumps of the eye in the act of reading. This again is an integration that can best be understood by assuming a hierarchy of informational levels.

The idea of hierarchy in vision is not easy to see, however, until one understands how intrinsic units are involved in the hierarchy and how the units of one level are combined to produce the units of higher levels. We are able to be quite specific about informational units at two different levels of the visual system. One of these is the most basic level, corresponding to the alphabet of printed English as an information-bearing system. This is the level of the nerve spike. Everything we know about the nerve spike makes it appear an appropriate manifestation of the most basic level of information transmission in the visual system. It is a discrete, discontinuous all-or-none phenomenon which has an invariant amplitude and invariant transmission characteristics under many circumstances. Thus, it is equivalent to the alphabetical letter or the dot or dash of telegraphic langauge. It is also an intrinsic natural unit which is not arbitrary, but which is natural to operation of the visual system. Even so, our knowledge of what sort of a code the information transmitted by a spike is put into is practically nil. In other words, we have a very vague conception of how a number of nerve spikes, in a number of related nerve fibers, are combined to convey different messages, such as the message, "This is an edge between dark and light with the light to the left." It is a mark of the slow movement of neurophysiology that such questions are only very gradually beginning to become considered more than

20 years after the solid foundations of information theory were laid. Since hundreds of receptor cells and nerve fibers are able to fire at once or nearly so, it should be noted that the problems of information transmission at this level have not only to do with seriality, as demonstrated in the analogy of chains of printed English, but also with parallel (i.e., nearly simultaneous) transmission. This is simply to say that another reason why the complexity of the visual systems has confounded us, is because in order to understand, we have to understand the peculiarities of a code that depends on the near-simultaneous occurrence of hundreds of events; whereas our reason is already taxed by the mere consideration of chains of single events. Even this says nothing of our lacking technical capacity to record from more than a few cells at a time.

After considering the lowest hierarchical level, represented by the nerve spike, we move to the consideration of higher hierarchical levels. It is virtually certain that the activity of many kinds of receptor ensembles and responding ensembles identified at various anatomical levels—retinal, lateral geniculate, and cortical—contain examples of intrinsic units. Thus, extensive neurophysiological studies of Hubel and Wiesel (1965), de Valois (1966), and many others have identified cells that respond to only a particular kind of stimulation such as a moving edge oriented in a particular direction or an "on" or an "off" light, etc. Although these cell ensembles, when taken as a whole, undoubtedly represent units at a higher hierarchical level than the nerve spike, their relationship to one another and to the natural process of vision is obscure. This can be made clearer by thinking of them as isolated words discovered in an unknown language. Although such words are intrinsically valid facts about the unknown language, they require interpretation to establish generalizations about the language. Thus, at this time these visual system units are important piece-meal facts waiting to be organized into an explanation.

Therefore, we must skip an unknown number of levels before we can positively identify another intrinsic unit in the informational hierarchy of the visual system. Then, however, we return to a familiar idea from earlier study (Secs. 2.3, 3.2, & 4.3): the informational package resulting from saccadic eye jumps. This, we argue, is the equivalent of a higher hierarchical level of printed English as a natural intrinsic informational unit of vision. It shares the common characteristics which have been delineated above, in that it: (a) divides the sensory material of the visual percept into intrinsic natural units (each unit corresponds to a new central fixation on a new area of the vision stimulus); (b) provides for greater complexity of the higher level of message by having greater length (in this case the greater length is in the dimension of time—the contrast between the fraction of a millisecond of the nerve spike versus the 50 to 1,000 milliseconds between eye jumps); (c) builds the higher unit (eye jump packages) out of chains of the lower units (nerve spikes as the lowest unit and response-specific cell ensembles responses at a higher level); (d) provides discontinuity in the structuring of the higher units out of the discontinuous lower units.

Discontinuity in the event that separates units has already been mentioned. The nerve spike is certainly a discontinuous phenomenon and we have shown in considerable detail how the all-or-none eye jump step function naturally packages visual information into units which are abruptly established by the displacement of the eye jump (Secs. 2.3, 3.2, & 4.5).

Chains of eye jump packages can easily be seen to occur—several are illustrated in the rows of circles of Figs. 4.6 and 4.7. Thus at the higher hierarchical level we are able to see chains. Likewise, at the level of nerve spikes we can see from any single-unit recording that chains have some meaning. However, until the codes which we have only cracked slightly at two levels are broken further, we cannot know more about these chains, which differ from the chains of printed English in not only having serial aspects but also aspects of parallel discharge. Thus seriality is only one aspect of visual information packaging. Because the nature of the coding is related to the fact that hundreds of receptor units and hundreds of nerve fibers fire together, parallel discharge as an important factor also results.

After seeing how the analogy to printed English fits further, we can better understand the issue of hierarchy in visual information handling. If one dealt merely with a point-for-point, one-for-one transformation of areas of the visual world to the retina to the brain where a photographic percept is formed, a nonhierarchical switchboard setup might work. However, when coding must be done at several levels and when information intake requires more than an instantaneous flash, the likelihood of a hierarchical structuring must be seriously entertained.

A final question we can examine further is the increase of complexity of information as one ascends the hierarchical scale. Here we are using the analogy to the types of messages that can be conveyed by different hierarchical levels—that an alphabetical letter can convey less complex information than a word, which in turn conveys less complex information than a sentence. Likewise, if we consider a nerve spike, the "meaning" of what it conveys would be analogous to an alphabetic letter—relatively meaningless in terms of complex structure and yet the building block of that structure. At a higher level, one would have coded messages such as "edge between green and red with the red to the left" (whose packaging we have not been able to specify). Again this message would in and of itself not be terribly meaningful. At a still higher level, the message of an eye jump package might be "an apple on a table (with colors and shapes specified)." Even higher, where several eye jumps are combined, would be the message "a still-life oil painting with an apple, a knife, a cheese, and a bottle on a table (with details and interrelationships specified)." As in the case of the structure of printed English we can see that this increased complexity has been achieved by increased "length" of message. This means that more time is required. A further understanding of the structure of visual perception may be gained by imagining this viewing of a painting takes place in the company of another person. After having looked at the painting, imagine that you next look at your companion. We now have a slightly higher level of complexity analogous to a chain of two sentences. Here the messages are of the form "organized percept of painting–organized percept of companion." There is a break between the two as you make the very long eye jump from the painting to the companion and lose the immediate detailed percept of the painting, and replace it by the immediate detailed percept of the companion. Here we are getting into matters we first considered in Sec. 1.7 and will examine further in Chap. 8. We are also at the edge of another issue which we will not be able to pursue here. This is the question of "action cycles" of behavior as elaborated by Calhoun, Spitz, and others (see Gaarder, 1966a for elementary discussion and references).

5.7. Recapitulation

We are now in a position to summarize and restate what we have found by drawing an analogy between printed English as an information-bearing system and the visual system as an information-bearing system. The first and most important point is that just as printed English and other languages have a hierarchical structure, so it appears we are impelled to assume a hierarchical structuring of increasing complexity in the information processing of the visual system. Thus, in order to dismiss our arguments, it must be positively shown that there are ways of structuring visual information which are not hierarchical, since we have generalized to assert that complex information-bearing systems are intrinsically and necessarily hierarchically organized. Assuming hierarchical organization, the next question is of intrinsic units. We have shown how the nerve spike corresponds to the basic unit–the alphabetic letter–and much of the book has been devoted to showing how the eye jump packages visual information into natural units at a higher level of the hierarchy. In doing this we have linked our work to other scientific quests for the discovery of intrinsic units which are natural to the phenomenon under study. The discontinuity of the units in visual perception is one of their simple properties—the nerve spike and the eye jumps are both abrupt, discrete, discontinuous phenomena. Likewise, the use of chains of lower units to form higher units is easily seen in the way that a chain of eye jump packages forms a higher unit of perception. The seriality of this is self-evident in spite of the fact that the simultaneous firing of many nerve spikes at once also makes parallel coding of spikes a certainty. We now have a model of the visual system which allows us to ask further questions about the relations between the visual system and other systems (Chap. 7), and will allow us to make a tentative model of behavior (Chap. 8). Before doing this, however, we will restate the complete model as it now exists (Chap. 6).

6 THE DISCONTINUOUS, FEEDBACK-MEDIATED, HIERARCHICAL, EDGE-INFORMATION PROCESSING MODEL OF VISION

6.1. Introduction

To this point, all of the necessary elements for a model of information processing by the visual system have been examined and discussed. While the resulting model will not be complete in the sense of totally explaining the visual process, it will be complete in the sense that what has been explained fits together and forms a connected whole. In this chapter we will list and briefly review the elements of the model (Sec. 6.2), and assemble them into the complete model (Sec. 6.3). Some of the ambiguities of the model as it presently exists will be presented followed by discussion of implications (Sec. 6.4) and criticisms of the model (Sec. 6.5).

6.2. Elements of the Model

We are now in a position to assemble the model of the visual system from the perspective chosen. Before doing this, we shall review the elements to be used in making the model. For the most part they will be in the order presented in the earlier chapters.

Feedback. Feedback is the concrete biological mechanism mediating homeostasis and adaptive control. In constructing our model of visual information processing, the essence of the role of feedback is that movement of the eyes through jumps and drifts of the eye is controlled in a way which in turn exerts control upon the resultant visual input. This is a feedback because the receptor system, which sends messages centrally is in turn altered by the eye movement, placing it in a new relationship to the visual environment. This has been explained in detail in Chap. 1 and in the simulations of Chap. 4.

Eye Jumps. A major feedback to the eye is attained through eye jumps. We have seen how eye jumps are also important in their own right as step functions which impose abrupt change upon the visual system and we have seen how this abrupt change is manifested by energy transformations in the occipital cortex, i.e., in the evoked response. We have further seen how the energy transformation can be considered as the overt manifestation of an information transformation. Reflecting upon the eye jump as a step function and utilizing the concrete insights provided us by computer technology, we can see how the eye jump causes the visual system to be a discontinuous processor. By use of analogies derived from simple photographic manipulations we can see how the visual system discontinuities cause the creation of informational packages which are manifested as edge templates during fixation and as massive transformations during larger eye jumps (Chap. 4). We can also see that the energy of evoked responses is a cortical manifestation reflecting in some way these eye jump informational packages (Chap. 2).

Eye Drifts and Tremor. The drift and tremor of the eye during eye fixation are another source of feedback. They are capable of providing continued changes of the edge information template during fixation pauses. These changes occur within the time boundaries of eye jumps and therefore constitute part of the eye jump package (Secs. 1.18 & 4.7).

Intrinsic Cortical Cycles. A recurrent discontinuous nervous phenomenon is by definition cyclical and represents an algorithmic chain with stochastic properties. Thus, certain events recur in an invariant sequence and other variable events recur in a variable sequence. Since some of these events take definite amounts of time, there are signs of periodicity, but since there is some variability of the amounts of time and since this variability has not been deciphered, periodicity often cannot be demonstrated (Chap. 3).

Information Organization. The cross-fertilization of information theory and visual physiology has led to further analysis of the organization of information. It can be shown that a number of information-bearing systems have the property of containing intrinsic informational units which are organized into hierarchies by time-dimensioned chains. On reviewing the visual system it is then found that a strong case can be made for the idea of eye jump packages representing discontinuous intrinsic units which are links in time-dimensioned chains and part of a hierarchy of informational organization (Chap. 5).

6.3. The Model

Here we will place together the elements of the model just reviewed and make from them a description of the model itself. Contrary to what we experience subjectively, and although the visual world itself may be continuous and may be reducible to simple nonhierarchical structure, we have analyzed facts about the visual system to show that eye jumps are crucial events which not only establish discontinuity in vision but also divide visual information into informational units which contain less than a simple one-for-one transformation of the visual world would contain (Secs. 1.13 & 5.6). The jump of the eye—not experienced with subjective awareness of the blur which would accompany it if there were not intervening mechanisms—results in an evoked response being generated, which in turn is the manifestation of a package of information being transmitted. Since the evoked response is an event with a self-limited, stereotyped time course, it may be assumed that the accompanying information is transmitted in similar ways—i.e., that it has a self-limited and stereotyped time course which puts it in the class of discontinuous processing mechanisms. We can also see that these events ordinarily occur on the order of one to four times a second. This means that they fit on the time scale between the nerve spike and alpha rhythm on the smaller side and the psychological unit of a second or two of time on the larger side (about the least amount of time with which we can subjectively deal without external stimuli to pace ourselves).

The energy package of the evoked response, which is identical with the informational package hypothesized, has a definite content. If the eye has just made a small fixation jump, the package contains a new set of edge templates. If the eye has just made a large jump, the package contains new sharply defined information about the new foveal contents, as well as containing a peripheral pattern which must be matched with the preceding fixation to obtain stabilization of the visual world.

Eye jump packages are of variable time durations—from 50 milliseconds to a second or two, and even much larger, as Steinman et al. (1967) have demonstrated under unusual circumstances. An eye jump package may be defined as the visual informational events occurring in the time between two eye jumps. The eye jump package has an invariable algorithmic temporal structure, the nature of which has not been completely analyzed, but which nevertheless can be described in some sequential features. Thus, the first event is the decision to make the eye jump. Next, the eye jump occurs with some kind of visual blanking during the event (see Secs. 2.7, 6.5, & 7.3).

Following the eye jump, an eye jump linked evoked response is generated and transmitted in the visual system, with the several transformations at neural junctions. Finally, the time domain of the period of fixation is entered. This complete cycle must be considered to represent not only a unit of information transmission, but also a temporal unit of short-term memory storage (see Sec. 7.2) since the short-term storage contents would be divided by the changes of information when eye jumps occur. Therefore, another subsequent part of the information package and of the short-term storage unit is the edge information template generated by the eye's drift during fixation and possibly by the tremor of the eye (see Sec. 4.7). Thus, we have shown that the eye jump package and the short-term memory storage consists of an invariant series: the eye jump generated edge information template contained in the evoked response followed by the edge information templates generated by drift and tremor. Whether both of these events or only one of them is crucial to perception has yet to be conclusively demonstrated. However, since either the eye jump generated component or the drift and tremor generated component can establish an information package, the model rests secure upon the fact that visual information is restructured by eye jumps.

These results of the eye jump have been carried on in harmony with the other activities of the brain, so that intrinsic cycles of brain activity, such as alpha, also provide clues as to how the pacing of vision is taking place. The model takes the facts pointing in this direction and from them assumes that brain cycles and eye movements are functioning in harmony as dual manifestations of the same underlying process.

This underlying process has to do with the organization of information by the brain. This means not only the organization of visual information, but information from all other sources as well, as we shall examine later (Chap. 8). As far as visual information is concerned, however, eye jumps serve to naturally divide it into units which are natural and intrinsic to the function of the brain and to its method of organizing information. In other words, the eye jump information packages are natural information-bearing packages of information which have their own place within a hierarchy of visual information-bearing structures. The eye jump packages are made of chains of nerve spike units with uncertain numbers of intervening hierarchic levels of units between. And the eye jump packages form chains of higher level units out of which the unit we may think of as a "percept" evolves.

The model can be schematically visualized (Fig. 6.1). The three components of the figure show: (*a*) furthest away, the EEG alpha as a reflection of

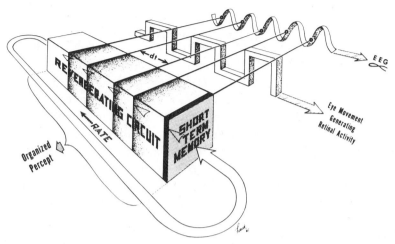

Fig. 6.1. Schematic model of eye jumps establishing successive separate templates of edge information reverberating through a storage cycle with a number of units. The near figure represents the circulation of templates within a short-term memory cycle. Present storage of past events recedes. The figure simulating eye movements emphasizes the discontinuity of eye jumps responsible for the discrete templates, while the EEG figure anticipates correlation between eye jumps, information processing and central nervous system events. (From "Mechanisms in Fixation Saccadic Eye Movements" by K. Gaarder, *British Journal of Physiological Optics,* 1967, **24,** 28–44. Reprinted by permission of the editors.)

intrinsic cycles; (*b*) in the middle, the step function eye jumps which generate retinal activity, causing evoked responses linked to the alpha; and (*c*) closest, central processes which reflect packaging, short-term memory storage, reverberating circuits as a possible mechanism of storage, the production of an organized percept, and the existence of a rate of package generation reflected in the rate of eye jumps. The packages can be visualized in the "blocks" making up the short-term memory. The content of the packages can be the eye jump linked evoked response generated edge templates, the drift generated template or both. The visualization is incomplete and is only meant to convey some of the major concepts of the model.

This then is our model—eye jumps interrupting and changing the visual input to establish informational packages which are natural units in the hierarchy of visual information organization.

6.4. Implications of the Model

Some major implications of the model will be discussed later in describing hypothetical alternatives for audiovisual interaction (Chap. 7) and for behavior in general (Chap. 8). A model that is able to detail mechanisms in one sensory system is bound to have implications for other sensory systems and for brain function in general. These, however, are outside of the sphere of vision, to which we will confine ourselves at this point.

Certain things have been left unsaid so far in the model that can be straightforwardly derived from it. One such thing has to do with the place implied for stochastic processes and entropy. Entropy is an informational measure which reflects the degree to which a given informational system fully utilizes its potentialities for variety. (It has been defined by Shannon [1948] as Entropy $= H = -\Sigma p_i \log p_i$; where p_i is the probability of one of a set of discrete events.) Thus, the entropy of the letters of a language of 26 letters which have an equal probability of occurrence would be greater than the entropy of English where the probabilities are highly constrained—i.e., where the probability of a letter being an e is much greater than the probability of a letter being a z. By the same token, the entropy of a set of fixation edge templates where the eye movement vectors have many directions and magnitudes is much greater than the entropy of a set of fixation edge templates where the eye movement vectors are homogeneous. Likewise, the entropy of a set of gross eye jump packages is greater if the jumps are between different parts of the same scene than if they concentrate on only a few elements of the scene. Further, the higher the rate of eye jumps, the greater the entropy. Informational entropy calculations upon biological data have not often been possible, and one of the immediate uses of our model is in the potential it provides for data analysis in terms of entropy.

The same physiological events used in our model are dealt with by Noton and Stark (1971a, 1971b) in a way complementary to this presentation. They see gross eye movements as resulting in serial presentation of visual input and conceptualize *feature rings* as a manifestation of a somewhat stereotyped typical scan path for any individual in examining a particular scene. While I have dealt very little with the ideas of learning and recognition, these are major issues in their model. Likewise, it would seem that certain issues which I go to great lengths to establish, for example discontinuity and hierarchy, may from their standpoint of engineering sophistication be taken for granted. Mayzner, Tresselt, and Helfer (1967) also have a similar model of visual input processing.

Our earlier treatment of homeostasis in vision (Sec. 1.11) was incomplete because it did not explain the homeostatic regulation of image processing. Having completed the model of vision, we now have a basis for describing the regulation of image processing. One aspect of the regulation is in the regulation of the rate of processing through control of the rate of eye jumps, referred to earlier (Sec. 3.3) and described in more detail later (Sec. 8.2). This is a fertile field for further work, since we have defined in rate of eye jumps a major dimension of visual attention. This is relatively easy to measure and offers a major new psychophysiological parameter. Work to date has mainly been scattered observations of unusual processing rates in specific situations. Thus, Hebbard and Fischer (1966) found striking increase in eye jumps during psychedelic states; Silverman and Gaarder (1967) found changed eye jump rates in schizophrenic patients; Gaarder (1967b) observed correlations between presence and absence of alpha and rate of eye jumps and between rate of eye jumps and the processing of speech. This later observation has also been made by Horn (1965).

Other aspects of regulation of image processing need to take into account the entropy of the stimulus versus the entropy of the processing. This awaits further conceptualization of the dimension of entropy in stimuli, but has been anticipated in a rudimentary way by studies of eye movements in relation to stimuli (Gaarder, 1960; Mackworth & Bruner, 1966; Mayzner et al., 1967; and Noton & Stark, 1971a, 1971b). A detailed analysis of image processing regulation requires further specific elaboration of the model, but the basis for doing so can be appreciated at this time.

Even though the model has been derived from experiments on the human visual system and described in terms of the human visual system, it appears certain that it will prove translatable to lower animals as well. As one small example, observation of birds and squirrels easily shows how their frequent abrupt head movements perform a function equivalent to eye jumps in the packaging of their visual information.

6.5. Criticisms of the Model

The model as presented can be critically evaluated from a number of points of view, some of which we can briefly consider. One of these concerns the scope of the model—how much it tries to explain and how much it fails to explain. Part of the value of a model is in its explanation of important issues. Another critical perspective has to do with whether a model explains what it sets out to explain. A more important question currently is whether a model fits the experimental facts as they are known. A more elusive question is whether a model is conceptually sound, whether or not its parts fit together logically. Implicit models organized around cryptic statements in the journal literature are especially liable to fall short on this point, because whole other realms of data are often ignored. A related question about a model is how much of it is valid and how much not. Sometimes the central concept of a model is valid even though the route to the concept is illogical, while other times the central concept is invalid, but the ordering of facts leads to the later discovery of new concepts. Even with a partly valid model, there is also the question of how much is new in what is valid.

It remains for time and scientific consensus to answer these general questions. An attempt has been made here to formulate a model ordering important facts concerning the visual system into a coherent picture of the visual process. How well the attempt has succeeded may not yet be clear. However, it is possible to raise a number of quite specific issues in relation to the model and consider some of the above questions with these issues. This will be done next.

Dynamic versus Static Models. Someday, when the controversy has been better resolved, an important chapter in the history of vision will concern man's many attempts to resolve the question of whether eye movements play an important role in vision. Although there are other dynamic models of vision, the important ones to date have been based on giving a crucial role to eye movements. Part of this history has been reviewed by Steinman et al. (1973). The history may be truncated by stating that although dynamic models have had intuitive appeal to many, they have consistently failed the test of being reducible to specific mechanisms experimentally demonstrable. Although this may be partly excused by the argument that the experiments were not well enough designed to make the test (see the reasoning of Worden reviewed in Sec. 1.14), nevertheless static models have dominated recently. (It is also worth pondering the fact that while intuition lead some to dynamic models, it just as surely leads others to static models.)

Some of these issues were considered in Chap. 1, where dynamic models can be considered the equivalent of feedback-mediated homeostatic models, while static models would be those in which there was no possibility of altering or selecting visual information at the receptor level. The terminology "dynamic" versus "static" predates the cybernetic engineering terminology of feedback and homeostasis. The most telling argument against dynamic models concerns eye movements and visibility, which we will consider next.

Eye Movements and Visibility. The most important findings here involve two facts: that vision fails with the stopped retinal image, but that visual fixation without eye jumps is possible. Both of these facts have been reviewed by Steinman et al. (1973) who have made major experimental contributions in this area. One approach to studying the stopped retinal image has been to reintroduce artificially the movements eliminated in the stopped image experiments. When this is done, it is found that neither the eye jump nor the tremor helps restore the visibility of the target as well as the drift (Alpern, 1972). This finding is further strengthened by the observation of Steinman et al. (1967) and others (see Steinman et al., 1973) that visual fixation without eye jumps is possible without apparent alteration of the visual percept. These facts lead to the major criticism of the model: If vision is possible without eye jumps, then eye jumps are not crucial to vision. This criticism was more telling in earlier version of the model (Gaarder, 1970), where a role for drift had not been assigned (see Secs. 4.7, 6.2 & 6.3). When drift-generated edge templates are considered as a possible component of eye jump packages, then long periods of fixation may be seen either as eye jump packages of unusually long duration or as periods in which some other mechanism of cortical intermittency intervenes to package the cortical input.

We must at this time decide the relative weight to give two contrasting lines of evidence: On the one hand, long periods without eye jumps are possible and eye jumps are not the most important component in restoring stopped image vision. On the other hand, gross eye jumps and fixation eye jumps are almost always present during vision, the eye jump evoked response exists, and eye jumps undoubtedly package input. These observations are most readily reconciled by assuming that our model as presented is valid, that a drift generated component to the eye jump package exists, and that the method of packaging during long interjump intervals remains uncertain. This does not seem to make the model too ambiguous or uncertain in view of the heavy weight of logical and experimental evidence presented thus far favoring it, since it is only the method of packaging in an unusual situation, not extensively studied, that is at issue.

Another crucial consideration is, that although fixation without eye jumps has been reported by Steinman's group and others, this finding has not yet been verified beyond all doubt by measuring the torsional component of eye movement as well as the horizontal and vertical. For technical reasons the torsional component of the eye movement is eliminated. It will certainly be a worthy experiment to go to the added trouble of measuring this component so that fixation without eye jumps can indeed be demonstrated beyond question. Even if fixation without eye jumps should be verified, the argument of Steinman et al. (1973) that this is a major type of eye movement pattern in visual information processing is not convincing and the overwhelming observation remains that most of the time the eye jumps about.

Suppression of Vision during Eye Jumps. A major area of recent research effort has been the deciphering of visual events occurring during eye jumps.

While numerous studies show some suppression of vision (see Alpern, 1972, and Steinman et al., 1973, for review), some others do not (Krauskopf, Graf, & Gaarder, 1966). The details of this issue are outside of the scope of the model presented here, which does not attempt to deal with the mechanisms of eye jumps. The major argument in support of the model is that whatever happens during eye jumps, there can be no question either logically or experimentally but that there is some kind of major transformation of visual information input, which is all that the model requires (see Sec. 7.3 for further clarification of this).

The Eye Jump Linked Evoked Response Represents the Blur during Eye Jumps. If the model did not include drift-generated edge template information in eye jump packages, the meaning of the eye jump linked evoked response would be crucial. As it is, however, this is not a crucial question. It should only be noted that to postulate the evoked response represents blur is to postulate that a major retinal and cortical response indistinguishable from the retinal and cortical response to flashed visual stimuli, which is associated with the perception of the flashed stimuli, represents wasted effort of the system. Again, as in the last paragraph, our argument would be that at the very least the evoked response represents a transformation dividing information into packages—the analog of the space between words or the period between sentences in the hierarchical structure of language (Sec. 5.4).

Edge Template Generation by Drifts versus by Eye Jumps. It could be argued that drift-generated edge templates are all that has been demonstrated, but these are what is already known anyway, so nothing new has been contributed. This criticism is a variant of the last and does not take into account the issues just considered—that eye jumps divide the temporal structure of the visual world by a major informational transformation.

Fixation Eye Jumps Are "Busy Work." This is a major conclusion of Steinman et al. (1973). This conclusion has apparently been reached by failing to recognize the importance of informational transformations in the hierarchical organization of information and when this factor is taken into account the crucial role of fixation eye jumps can be easily seen. Since eye jumps transform the temporal chain of visual input, they divide that input into natural units de facto.

Periodicity Has Not Been Shown. The downfall of many previous attempts at demonstrating cortical excitability cycles has been the failure to demonstrate periodicity. This is based on equating the existence of a cycle with precise temporal periodicity, whereas the major feature of most biological phenomena is that cycles occur in which the time in some steps of the cycle (i.e., link in the chain) is variable from one cycle to the next. The idea of cycles with many invariant steps has an overwhelming logical force once the idea has been released from the constraint of periodicity.

Issues Not Considered in the Model. Many important issues are not dealt with by the model, but have not been considered crucial to the model. These will be briefly reviewed in relation to the model.

1. *Voluntary versus involuntary control of eye movements.* Steinman et al. (1973) have presented and reviewed compelling arguments that large and small eye jumps are both voluntary and are under the same control. This is consistent with the model.

2. *Slow control of the eye during fixation.* The same group has also argued well for the idea that eye fixation is maintained by slow control. Since the slow control requires a visible target, it is a feedback control. Therefore the drift-generated edge templates may be considered under feedback control, consistent with the model.

3. *Eye jumps as an overlearned mechanism.* Steinman et al. (1973) make use of the concept of overlearning to partly account for the "busy work" of fixation eye jumps. It is well to recognize that the concept of overlearning is a shorthand simplification of a complicated process, seeming to explain more than it really does in a circular chain of reasoning.

4. *Eye jumps as a scanning mechanism.* The concept of scanning is borrowed from engineering technology but is usually not well defined. The analogy is not strong between the single scanning spot of a television screen and the simultaneous sweeping across all retinal receptors during an eye jump. Scanning models must say *exactly* what they mean by scanning.

5. *Feedback mechanisms versus feedforward mechanisms and stability of the visual world.* Stability of the visual world is a recognized fact accounted for by various theories. Some of these theories postulate ideas of feedback (Skavenski, 1972) and feedforward (von Holst, 1954). Although the reasoning of these theories is close and derived from several disciplines (see Matin, 1972), the idea of feedforward is probably related to positive feedback and to homeokinesis.

Ultimately, it is for the reader to evaluate the model, these criticisms of the model, and others he may discern. Likewise, it is for scientific consensus, arrived at through experiment and reasoning, to decide the fate of the model.

6.6. Recapitulation

In this chapter the complete model is presented. The model of visual information processing uses the elements of feedback, eye jumps, eye drifts and tremor, intrinsic cortical cycles, and information organization in hierarchy. These elements are combined into a model wherein visual information is hierarchically organized by eye jumps, which package the information into natural units. Some implications of the model are examined and some criticisms of the model are presented and answered.

7 AUDIOVISUAL INTERACTION—THE PROGRAMMING OF DIFFERENT SENSORY INPUTS

7.1. Introduction

In this chapter we shall examine alternatives for explaining the way in which sensory input from different sensory modalities interact in the brain. The concept of interaction explains issues similar to those explained by the concept of input programming. The concepts differ, since the older idea of interaction implies the action of one modality *upon* the other—i.e., how hearing might affect vision—while the newer concept of input programming concerns the somewhat more restricted question of how each of the modalities is processed by the brain relative to the others.

Sensory modalities include sight, hearing, taste, touch, and smell. These senses are considered exteroceptive, since they are used to perceive things outside (exterior to) the body. It is also reasonable to include the interoceptive (inside the body) senses, such as position sense, deep pain sense, gut sensations, etc., as well. The relationship between the senses, memory, and current thought is a further question which will be considered in Chap. 8.

In the rest of this chapter we will focus our attention on two sense modalities—sight and hearing. We will assume that a similar scheme may account for interactions between other sensory modalities not considered. In other words, if we can come up with a reasonable picture of audiovisual information processing, we can see that the same kind of an interactive system, or at least one that deals with the same issues, may account for wider interactions—such as the interaction between the visual system and touch or between the sensory processing of one's own respiratory pattern and the position sense in one's limbs. Finally, in Chap. 8, we will find ourselves in a position to consider some important alternatives for a general model of behavior which is derived from the study of sensory interaction—we will be able to draw tentative conclusions about the interaction of the major components of the nervous system.

In this chapter, however, we will simplify our field by considering only the auditory and the visual systems. To do this we will: (*a*) Recapitulate the idea of discontinuity in the visual system in a simplified way which fits the arguments to be constructed (Secs. 7.2 & 7.3). (*b*) Show how a similar concept can be applied to the auditory system (Sec. 7.4). (*c*) Use these concepts to define possible alternative methods of input programming given what we know about input (Sec. 7.5).

7.2. Schematizing Visual Input Discontinuity

In earlier sections (Secs. 1.19, 2.3, 3.2, 4.2-4.5, 5.3, 5.6, & 6.5), extensive justifications were given for considering visual input as discontinuous. In this chapter we shall continue this line of reasoning and use schematic presentations to show what is happening at the same time in both the auditory and visual systems. In order to achieve familiarity with this new method of notation we will now restate the idea of visual system discontinuity using this schema.

In this notation, borrowed from digital circuit technology and oscilloscope test procedures, a horizontal line is used to depict certain events by an abrupt vertical jump of the line. This is a step function with two positions, one of which is the occurrence of the event, the other of which is the nonoccurrence of the same event. For example, if we consider the eye jump system, we can say that there are two events—an eye jump is occurring or it is not occurring. This is shown in Fig. 7.1. The line in its lower horizontal position represents no eye jump occurring, while the jumping of the line to the upper position happens when an eye jump occurs and the line stays in the upper position

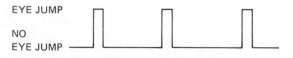

Fig. 7.1. Schematic notation of eye jumps.

until the eye jump is completed. The horizontal dimension represents time, and its units will be considered arbitrary. By arranging a number of these schemata in a column it is possible to show what is occurring in several systems simultaneously. It should be noted, so as to avoid confusion, that these representations may be of actual or hypothetical events. Those readers who are experienced with oscilloscopes will readily see that our schematic notation is analogous to the horizontal traces of the oscilloscope screen when step functions are applied at the input.

In the next figure (Fig. 7.2), we shall use the schematic notation to show what is happening simultaneously in two systems—an "actual" system of simulated eye jumps and a hypothetical system which represents the discontinuous input processing discussed earlier (Secs. 4.5, 5.6, & 6.3). The upper trace represents the same eye jumps just considered, while the lower trace represents a hypothetical visual information input, with the trace being in the lower position when no input is being taken in and in the upper position when input is being taken in. As explained earlier, the mechanism hypothesized is that a rapid shift of the retinal image presents a changed new image after the shift has been completed which is taken in as an evoked response package carrying the new information put on the new retinal image.

The schematization is also useful because it helps us to see some of the limitations of the word pictures we have painted so far. One such limitation is that we have not dealt thoroughly with the questions of exactly how long visual information is taken in and exactly when the information is taken in, relative to an eye jump. The schematic notation has forced a decision on both these questions in order to make the drawing. We have arbitrarily drawn Fig. 7.2 to show that the moment visual input begins is the same moment the eye jump finishes. It might instead be 10 milliseconds later, or it might be just before an eye jump, or it might have another relationship. Since we do not know, we have had to assume. Likewise, we must designate an arbitrary

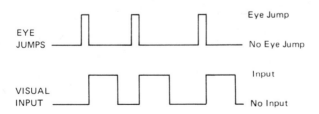

Fig. 7.2. Schematic notation of eye jumps and discontinuous input processing.

length of time during which visual input takes place. These ambiguities of the word pictures have been arbitrarily resolved here by making assumptions to which we are forced in using the schematic notation. However, since we do not have a solid basis for the assumptions, it must be remembered that the assumptions are arbitrary. Nevertheless, we can see that there are a limited number of discrete alternatives and that we gain by making such tentative distinctions and reserving final judgment until more facts are known.

Although we have created a notational system for certain events, we have not thereby been able to tell where these events take place. Since the early components of evoked responses seems to reach the cortex without great temporal variability and since there are several variable waves to the later response, it may be that these events of timing occur in the cortex.

Another issue demanding clarification is raised by our schematic representations also. This is the question of what happens to visual events which take place during a non-input moment. We can show this in Fig. 7.3 by adding a third line which we will call "external stimuli" where there are three "events" designated A, B, and C. We can assume they are identical brief flashes of light equal in location and intensity. Notice that Event A occurs during a moment of visual input. We would, therefore, assume it would be perceived. Notice that Event B occurs during an eye jump. From studies of visual threshold during eye jumps (Steinman et al., 1973; Zuber & Stark, 1966) we would assume that it might or might not be perceived, depending on the size of the eye jump and the intensity of the stimulus, among other things. Event C occurs during neither an eye jump nor a moment of visual input. Would it be perceived? Extensive observations by many investigators have shown that appreciable numbers of brief flashes well above threshold do not routinely disappear, so we must conclude that events which occur during non-input

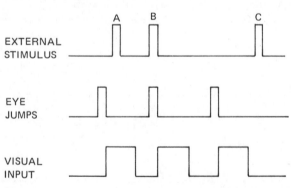

Fig. 7.3. Possible relations between external stimuli and input moments.

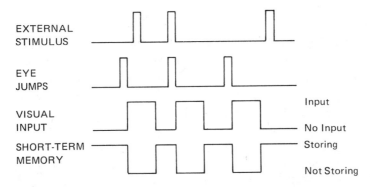

Fig. 7.4. Schematic notation of short-term memory and input moments.

moments are not lost. The current explanation for this is that there is short-term memory (Averbach & Sperling, 1961; John, 1972). Again, this concept has been made concrete by computer technology, just as with the distinction between the continuous and discontinuous (Secs. 2.3 & 4.2). We can designate short-term memory in our schematic notation by adding a fourth line to Fig. 7.3 to get Fig. 7.4 which shows a short-term memory as the mirror image of the visual input—when visual input is open the short-term memory is "dumping out" its contents into visual input, while when visual input is closed, the short-term memory is open to sensory impressions and is storing external stimuli to be held until the next input moment. Although there is extensive recent work studying short-term visual memory and short-term memory in other systems, it is beyond our scope to consider it further here. A review of the subject is in Jameson and Hurvich (1972).

7.3. Vision during Eye Jumps

While using schematic notation to explain visual input processes in greater detail we can produce a further argument favoring the idea of visual input discontinuity. This will counter the implicit common sense assumption that visual information input is intrinsically continuous in its nature. Schematic notation offers another way to show that even when visual input is assumed continuous, its informational nature is still discontinuous. This may be seen by recalling that when continuous visual information transmission is assumed, it must also be assumed that the retinal image information transmitted during an eye jump is that of a blurred or smeared image. We may take "blurred" or "smeared" to mean that nonuseful information or noise is transmitted. As the only other remote alternative, the retinal image information during an eye jump, might be transformed into a type of information in which each retinal element transmits information about the successive parts of the retinal image that sweep across it. We raise this remote explanation to consider all logical possibilities and still have as the only conclusion that information transmitted during an eye jump is markedly different from information transmitted during moments of visual fixation. In other words, there are at least two states of information transmission in the visual system. One can be called "transmission during fixation" (designated "F" for fixation) and the other can be called "transmission during eye jumps" (designated "B" for blur). Transmission during eye jumps is either blurred or inhibited or of a drastically different nature than transmission during fixation. In schematic notation, this results in Fig. 7.5.

Assuming continuous visual processing, we still have interruptions caused by eye jumps resulting in discontinuous informational input of the form: FBFBFBFBFB . . . . In other words, even if the receptors were continuous transmitters, and there were no memory storage where information was held, the effect of the eye jump upon the retinal image still makes the visual system a discontinuous information processing system. The only exception to this is vision during fixation where there are long periods with no eye jumps (see Steinman et al., 1973). Here intervals between saccades may be many seconds long. Among alternatives raised by this finding are the possibility of recirculation of a short-term memory package representing a form of idetic imagery or the possibility that visual input is not solely controlled by eye jumps but that other "shutters" or "gates" or methods of packaging operate as well (Sec. 6.5). Some explanation is also necessary to account for the

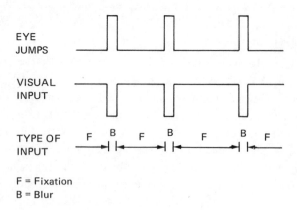

F = Fixation
B = Blur

Fig. 7.5. Schematization of vision during eye jumps illustrating discontinuity even in the most extreme case.

relationship between eye jump linked evoked responses and its accompanying edge information template, drift-generated templates, short-term storage, and input moments. However, it is not necessary to completely specify these relationships in order to use the models.

7.4. Auditory Information Input

If discontinuity of visual information processing is not readily comprehended, the idea of discontinuity of auditory processing is even less comprehensible. Again, one reason is that there is little subjective basis for assuming discontinuity—the stream of auditory consciousness is just as readily experienced as strictly continuous as is the stream of visual consciousness. Indeed, the very idea of a stream implies continuity (see James [1950] on the stream of consciousness). For the scientifically trained, the awareness of sound waves as the tangible physical basis of hearing also implies continuity. In thinking of waves, one does not conceive simultaneously of the idea of the waves being broken up into discontinuous packaging.

Nevertheless, again there is a basis for assuming things are not as they appear, and that hearing, as well as vision, involves discontinuity. One major basis for this assumption is that much experimental work has shown that it is not possible for the auditory system to make the discrimination of which of two events is the first if they occur sufficiently close to one another. Thus, if two very brief clicks which can be discriminated by amplitude or pitch are presented to a subject sufficiently close to one another in time (say 25 milliseconds apart), the subject cannot tell which of the two came first (Hirsch, 1959). This is most obviously interpreted to mean that the two clicks are both taken into the same short-term memory storage bin, where the discrimination of successiveness (i.e., which came first), is not made and that the two clicks are then "read into" consciousness (or into a "processor") without temporal discrimination as to which came first (White, 1963). Other more complex evidence has also been interpreted to mean the same thing (Hirsch, 1959), but we will not go into that here.

Although in the visual system rather straightforward mechanisms for dividing information into packages can be readily hypothesized and studied in eye jump feedback, no such marker has been identified in the auditory system. There is yet almost no way, outside of short offhand experiments during neurosurgery, to examine what is going on in the ear of man during hearing. Not only is experimentation more difficult, but the very nature of auditory information as opposed to visual information further complicates the situation. Thus, whereas prototypes of visual information processing are the moving eye gazing over a stationary visual environment or reading written text, a prototype of auditory information processing might be listening to speech. It can be seen, in vision of the sorts described, that a feedback which is controlled by the organism and directed toward formal aspects of the stimulus organization such as the written lines, would adequately allow processing of different parts of the scene. On the other hand, in listening to speech it seems likely that the kind of information processing which would be optimal would be to divide the input into units whose nature was determined in part by the input. In other words, speech would most naturally be divided into units according to the nature of the speech itself, rather than having the processor divide the speech in a way arbitrary to the speech's own nature; the latter would seem to be the case if an auditory nerve feedback were being used to process the speech. This is only a small example of how the study of two sense modalities requires constant attention to the question of whether to generalize between the two modalities and assume the same mechanisms operative or whether to pay attention to intrinsic differences in the nature of the information to be processed by the different modalities and look for different mechanisms. Further, whereas in the visual system we have a good understanding of the physiological and informational nature of units at the level of the eye jump package, in the auditory system the same questions are almost completely obscure.

Pilot study has been made of this question by eliciting evoked responses to a tape loop of spoken words which repeated every few seconds (Gaarder, unpublished study). The main outcome of this study was to demonstrate the necessity to ensure that the stimulus retains its novelty to prevent the subject from immediately habituating to the monotonous stimulus. If habituation were prevented, the nature of auditory unit packaging might be deduced. One likely possibility is that the packaging is done by the listener using feedback to "lock on" to the rhythm of the speaker (Worden, 1966). Much work by the kinesic school has shown that when a speaker and a listener converse there is a "dance" going on between them in which the listener picks up a rhythm from the speaker and keeps time with it. The reality of this is demonstrated by the slow motion analysis of motion pictures which pick up the bodily movements of both speaker and listener (Birdwhistell, 1970). The fact that telephone communication is possible where the speaker is not seen can be explained by assuming the voice carries the same rhythm to lock onto that is carried more thoroughly by bodily movements—that a listener picks up a speech rhythm which he locks onto and thereby imitates. He would use clues in the rhythm to indicate how and when he wishes to package the input by reading it out of storage. Thus, for instance, he might read out of storage on every beat of the rhythm. Interesting clues to this also come from analysis of eye movements during listening (Gaarder, 1967b, 1969; Horn, 1965), where it is shown that some listeners have a striking increase in rate of eye movements while they listen as compared to silent epochs.

To summarize what is known about discontinuity of auditory perceptions, we can say there is strong presumptive evidence to assume it is operative, but there is little information on how auditory input is divided into intrinsic information-bearing units—whether the control is from inside by a feedback or whether the control is from outside by a registration of intrinsic characteristics of the input which cause it to be broken up into units based on its own properties, or whether some combination of these two exists.

7.5. Models of Auditory-Visual Interaction

The next task is to spell out assumptions from which we will derive a model of audiovisual interaction and then consider alternative models and an experiment for choosing between them. First, we will assume information processing is hierarchically organized in both the visual and the auditory system. We will then assume nearly identical properties for both systems at two levels. At one level we assume the nerve spike is the basic unit of coding. At the other level we assume both systems have discontinuity of their processing somewhere in the 50- to 500-millisecond time range. Based on earlier consideration of the organization of information (Chap. 5), we will further assume that this discontinuity will divide the input into units which are intrinsic to the informational coding of the processor. While we have shown how this is true of the visual system, we have also made a good case for the idea that information-bearing hierarchies are naturally divided into chains of intrinsic units. Therefore, we have a basis for expecting the same property in the auditory system.

From these assumptions we can return to schematic notations (Sec. 7.2) to see how there are several ways in which the auditory and visual system might process input. Alternative models are strictly limited to three, which are serial, parallel, or independent. These are schematized in Figs. 7.6 (serial), 7.7 (parallel), and 7.8 (independent). Serial sensory input is characterized by the fact that processing of one modality automatically excludes the processing of another. Thus, in Fig. 7.6, when the visual "gate" is open, the auditory "gate" is always closed; and conversely when the auditory "gate" is open, the visual "gate" is always closed. Parallel processing means that when either the visual "gate" or the auditory "gate" is open the other is also always open

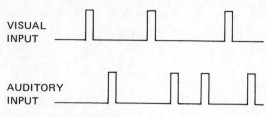

Fig. 7.6. Serial processing.

(Fig. 7.7). Independent processing means that whether one system was processing or not had nothing to do with whether the other system is processing (Fig. 7.8).

We can again notice how schematic diagrams reveal the imprecision in word pictures. Thus, in diagramming serial processing we have been forced to choose between having times when both gates are closed versus having one gate open at all times. We have chosen to have times when both gates are closed because this allows the model to be expanded to include serial processing of other sense modalities, whereas if one of two gates was always open, then a third input could not also be processed serially.

Having a set of hypothetical alternative models, we may now choose between them by experimentation. We may best understand how such an experiment might be constructed by first considering the effect of an input "moment" upon the subsequent reaction time to a stimulus taken in during the moment of input. We will show how total reaction time is dependent upon the time between the stimulus occurring and the input moment occurring. This can again best be understood from diagrams. Figure 7.9 shows two alternative input situations and the resulting reaction times. In Fig. 7.9A, a stimulus occurs a long time before an input moment and in Fig. 7.9B, the stimulus occurs at the same time as the input moment occurs. The result of these alternatives is that in "A" the reaction time is longer than in "B" by the

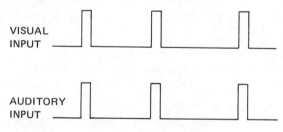

Fig. 7.7. Parallel processing.

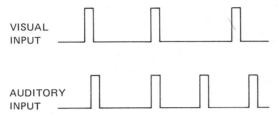

VISUAL
INPUT

AUDITORY
INPUT

Fig. 7.8.   Independent processing.

amount of time the stimulus in "A" has to wait for the input moment to occur. This conclusion is arrived at by assuming an identical mean central processing time in both cases. The mean central processing time is the time it takes the stimulus to be processed and result in an output of a reaction time, *once taken in* through the input gate at the input moment. Since in "A" the stimulus must wait for the moment to occur, while in "B" the moment is already there, the reaction time in "A" is longer by the amount of time which must pass until the moment occurs.

It may be noted here that we are also helping to account for the well-known variability of individual reaction times by assuming there is a component of that variability which is caused by having to wait variable periods for the input moment to occur when the stimulus is applied. By further assuming that there are output moments as well as input moments, one would be able to completely account for individual reaction times by three determining factors: (*a*) the time to wait for an input moment to occur; (*b*) having to wait a variable number of central periods until an output moment occurs; and (*c*) the length of the periods during the epoch. The length of periods during the epoch might still be determined by further intangibles, however, leaving a residual unaccounted variability.

This explains how the relation between the time of occurrence of the stimulus and the time of occurrence of the input moment affects the reaction time. This allows us to set up an experiment in which we will indirectly control the moment at which stimuli are presented in relation to the input moment and subsequently analyze reaction times to determine the nature of the relation between moment of stimulus presentation and input moment. This may be done by locking the auditory stimulus to the visual input moment with a fixed delay. Assuming the visual moment has a relation to the auditory moment, the stimulus is then related to the auditory moment. Since we will be using a signal related to the visual input moment to determine the moment of auditory stimulus presentation, this allows us to deduce the

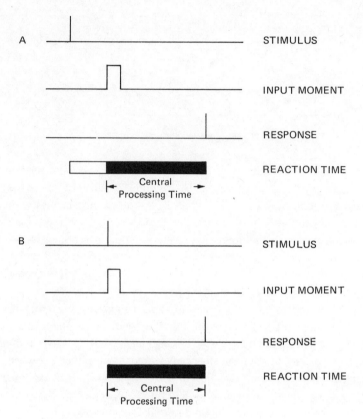

Fig. 7.9. Illustration of the effect upon a subsequent reaction time of when a stimulus is given relative to an input moment. In A, the stimulus is given before an input moment and there is an additional component to the reaction time as compared to B, where the stimulus is given during an input moment.

relationship between auditory and visual input moments. This will then allow us to make a choice between the three alternative models of sensory interaction—the serial, the parallel, and the independent (Figs. 7.6, 7.7, and 7.8).

In order to understand the experiment further, we will reconstruct Figs. 7.6, 7.7, and 7.8, adding in an auditory stimulus which will be controlled by an eye jump, and adding in a hypothetical reaction time. We will see how the relation between a given stimulus and the auditory input moment will be different in each model and how, thereby, the actual experimental results may help us to decide which model is the correct one. Figure 7.10 shows how

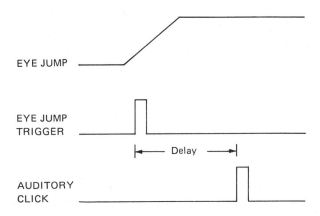

Fig. 7.10. Illustration of how the auditory stimulus is time locked to the eye jump with a fixed delay.

the eye jump may be used to trigger an eye jump trigger, as already explained (Sec. 2.5), and how the eye jump trigger may subsequently trigger an auditory click with a controlled time delay after the trigger signal. This is a relatively simple problem in electronic technology. Having equipment to carry out such a process, one may then test different stimulus time delays after an eye jump to see their effect on auditory processing. This may be done by considering four stimuli: One which occurs as soon after the eye jump begins as the trigger will allow, one which occurs at the end of the eye jump, one which occurs soon after the end of the eye jump, and one which occurs longer after the end of the eye jump. These alternatives are schematized on the left column of Fig. 7.11. We have changed our idealized schematic notation slightly by making the eye jump a slope instead of a perfectly vertical step function. This merely reflects that the eye jump, as with any step function, takes time to occur and that when the time scale is sufficiently expanded it will show a step function occurring over time rather than instantaneously. The time it takes a fixation eye jump to occur is between 5 and 15 milliseconds. The sloping part of the eye jump may be taken to represent this amount of time, although an exact time scale is not designated.

We have chosen four idealized stimulus times for the particular reason that they can be expected to have definite different relations to the auditory input moments in our three different models of sensory interaction (serial, parallel, and independent). These different relations can be conceptualized in relation to the visual input gate as follows:

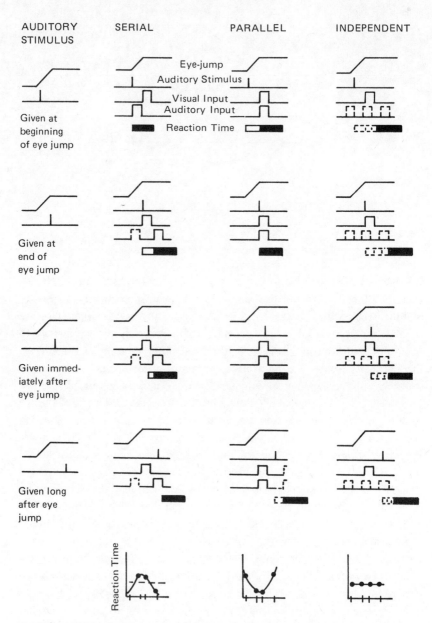

Fig. 7.11. Models of auditory-visual interaction. Idealized simulations of the effect of auditory stimuli with particular time delays relative to eye jumps with three hypothetical models of processing—serial, parallel, and independent.

1. A stimulus given during an eye jump would be expected to arrive before the visual input moment occurred, since the general finding of inhibition during eye jumps leads us to assume this to be the most likely period for the visual input *not* to occur.

2. A stimulus given at the end of an eye jump would arrive just as the visual input moment began, according to the model of discontinuous processing (Chap. 6).

3. A stimulus given soon after the end of an eye jump would also arrive during the visual input moment (which is assumed to have finite duration even though termed "moment").

4. A stimulus given longer after the end of the eye jump would arrive after the visual input moment and would not be part of that particular moment.

These four alternatives are pictured for the eye jump and the auditory stimulus in the left column of Fig. 7.11.

We have now visualized the eye jump, the auditory stimulus, and the assumed moment of visual input at the end of the eye jump. The remaining elements to be considered are the auditory input moment, the reaction time, and the components of the reaction time. The auditory input moment must be pictured in three different ways to account for the three different models of sensory interaction. This can be seen at the top of Fig. 7.11. *Parallel* processing is represented by the visual and auditory input moments occurring simultaneously and *independent* processing by the auditory input moments bearing no fixed relation to the visual input moments. *Serial* processing is arbitrarily represented as having the auditory moments on both sides of the visual moment. There are other possibilities for serial processing which are not considered. In Chap. 8 reasons will be given why, in an auditory task with heightened auditory attention, there might be a high density of auditory moments which serves to justify our particular notation of having auditory moments on both sides of the visual moment.

By considering the three models with the four time relations between visual input moment and stimulus, we have twelve possible outcomes of reaction time. Fig. 7.11 shows these and shows how in each case the reaction time would be affected by having to wait or not having to wait for an auditory input moment before the stimulus could be processed. We can examine each of these cases in turn to explain the outcome for that case and then draw curves to describe the reaction times in each model.

First, we will consider the *serial processing model*. If the auditory input stimulus is given just after the onset of the eye jump, it will be given before the visual input moment. Therefore, it will be given at a time which could be an auditory input moment and thus the reaction time will not include waiting for the auditory input moment to occur. Thus, the reaction time would be less than the mean reaction time, which must include both times of waiting and times of not waiting. If the auditory input stimulus is given just as the eye jump ends, it will occur just as the visual input moment begins. Therefore, there will be the maximum time to wait until the next auditory moment may begin, since in the serial model the visual and auditory moments may not coincide. Thus, the reaction time includes a long wait for the next input moment and being the longest reaction time would also be longer than the mean reaction time. If the auditory stimulus occurs after the end of the eye jump, there would be less and less time to wait for the end of the visual input moment and the possibility of an auditory input moment and consequently there would be a lessening of the reaction time and a lessening of the component of the reaction time due to waiting for the auditory input moment. The serial model curve shows these effects in the ∩-shape depiciting each of the four points explained above.

The outcome of a *parallel processing model* can be considered next. Here the visual and the auditory input moments coincide. Therefore, a stimulus given at the beginning of an eye jump must wait for the eye jump to end before the visual and auditory input moments occur. This causes the reaction time to be longer by the amount of time necessary for this to occur and, therefore, causes a reaction time greater than the mean reaction time and greater than the minimal reaction time. On the other hand, if the auditory stimulus is given at the end of the eye jump or soon after, this is during the visual and auditory input moments and it, therefore, has no wait before central processing. This leads to a minimum reaction time with no waiting for an input moment, and is less than the mean reaction time. Finally, a stimulus, given long after the end of the eye jump, occurs after the end of the visual and auditory input moment and requires a wait for the next input moment before it can be processed. Therefore, the reaction time would include a large component of waiting for the input moment, making it longer than the mean reaction time. The parallel processing curve shows these relations as a ∪-shaped curve.

Finally, the independent processing model is one in which the occurrence of an auditory input moment bears no relationship to the visual input moments. This is depicted by auditory input moments with no set relation to the visual input moment. Here, obviously, no matter what relation existed between the auditory stimulus and the eye jump, the relation time would not be affected, because the auditory input moments occur independent of the eye jumps and the visual input moments. Thus, the reaction time at any moment relative to the eye jump is the same as any other and the curve is a straight line depiciting the mean reaction time.

More complete details of an experiment which tests these alternatives are given elsewhere (Gaarder, 1969). The results may be summarized by saying that an independent processing model is tentatively excluded and that a ∩-shaped curve is found which favors a serial processing model. Although the evidence is inconclusive because of inherent difficulties in the experiment (see Gaarder, 1969), how to clearly decide between alternatives is plainly spelled out for future work.

A specific model if proven valid allows for numerous neurophysiological experiments to determine the sites of the time delays. Thus, there appear the major possibilities that serial sensory input to the central processor is either controlled at the thalamic and geniculate nuclei or within the cortex itself. These alternatives are readily testable in experiment. Schmidt and Kristofferson (1963) have other evidence which also supports a serial model.

7.6. Recapitulation

In previous chapters a basis has been laid for a model of visual information processing being organized with discontinuous hierarchically structured informational units accepted for central nervous system processing at input moments. Here arguments are presented for this, providing the means of modeling the interaction or programming of several sensory modalities. In particular, an experimental basis is described for differentiating between different methods of auditory-visual input processing. Possible methods are serial, parallel, or independent. The different effects of these different types of input processing upon reaction times are described and on the basis of experimental evidence it is tentatively concluded that audiovisual input is serially processed.

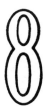 # A GENERAL MODEL OF BEHAVIOR

8.1. Introduction

Chapters 1, 2, and 3 laid out ideas about vision based on experimental evidence and logic to arrive at a specific and concrete model of discontinuous visual information processing linked with eye jumps. This model was described in Chap. 4 and combined in Chap. 5 with further compelling ideas about the organization of information in hierarchies to arrive at a fairly complete model of the visual process presented in Chap. 6. To that point in the description, the ideas dealt with were clear and the conclusions inescapable within the scope of the particular evidence considered.

The model represents a new way of considering the visual system. Psychological sciences often overlook the fact that a new view of a particular element of behavior may have inescapable broader implications for the overall understanding of the organism. In other words, one cannot usually reorganize a part without considering its effect upon the organization of the whole. Thus, in having imposed the idea of discontinuity of information processing upon the visual system, it was necessary to examine sensory interaction between the auditory and visual systems in Chap. 7. While the experimental evidence reported was equivocal, choices had to be made between serial, parallel, and independent processing models. There was then reason to favor the idea of serial processing between the auditory and visual systems. Through Chap. 6 solid evidence was offered, but in Chap. 7 the conclusions could not be certain.

Although the evidence was not airtight so that the choice was uncertain, just making the choice was good illustration of how that choice influences the overall model of behavior ultimately arrived at.

In this chapter we shall continue our argument that "if such and such is true then so and so must follow." To this purpose I shall show that if a bimodality serial processing model is valid, then many unsolved questions about behavior in general fall into place in terms of the model, and a general cybernetic model of behavior based on serial processing of all sense modalities emerges. This model considers cognitive and memory functions, too. The general model is presented as a speculation and is not meant to be given the same weight as the model of visual information processing. However, it is important to understand that even if a serial processing model is incorrect, the method has led to choosing among a limited number of alternatives, thereby acknowledging the issue that *some* model of behavior must be established in order to understand the behaviors under study. Thus, the hope is not so much that this model is entirely correct as that the alternatives that can be tested and chosen among have been indicated, and that from this choice important consequences may follow.

Modern engineering technology uses a similar method when all known methods of solving each step of a problem are put together in all possible combinations. Subsequently, the combinations which obviously won't work are eliminated, and further effort is put into the elaboration of the most promising of the remainder. This method was used in developing the jet engine, where all known methods of carrying out each step necessary to the final process were combined; those that obviously would not work were eliminated, and those that were most promising were followed. Therefore the correct model must at least be chosen from a small set of alternatives suggested by the model.

8.2. General Serial Model of Sensation

The leap is quite short from assuming that vision and hearing must be serially processed to hypothesizing that all sensory modalities must be serially processed. Such a model merely puts all other sense modalities under the same constraint that no two may be centrally processed at the same time, in other words, they may not share the same input moment. Once this has been done, certain things such as the question of selective sensory attention, become easy to explain.

These matters become clearest by the use of examples. In making generalizations from the two systems of vision and hearing, it is useful not to complicate things too much initially. Therefore, only two more sensory systems—smell and proprioception will be added. The classification of systems as it presently exists is not necessarily adequate. We do not know, for certain, exactly what things are covered in the category of proprioceptive input moments. Just limb position? Or do such things as limb movement and velocity also belong in this particular system? Are they processed separately? This will not necessarily affect our example adversely. Figure 8.1 shows a general model of sensory input processing, with the four modalities. It can be seen that each modality may have a rate of processing—its input moments may occur a certain number of times a second. It also will be seen that for the entire sensory system taken as a whole there is likewise a rate of processing. The major constraint upon the processing is that no two modalities may have the same input moment, since this is a serial processing model.

In order to see how the model helps in understanding selective attention, some examples which emphasize different sense modalities will be considered: every day events such as reading a book, relaxing while listening to music, sniffing a cooking broth, tying one's shoes in the dark, and watching television. The first four are chosen as relatively pure illustrations of using a particular sensory modality; the last (watching TV), shows the much more common compound activity, where several modalities are intimately related to one another in the activity.

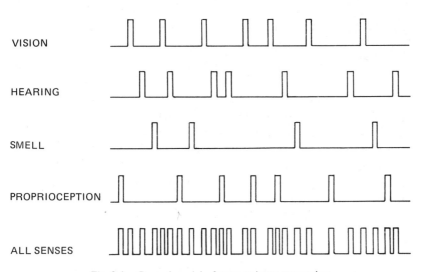

Fig. 8.1. General model of sensory input processing.

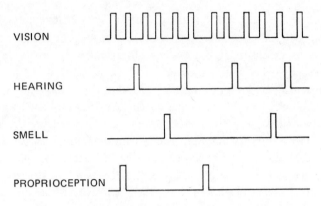

Fig. 8.2. Model of sensory input, processing while reading a book.

Figure 8.2 shows the input moments in the various modalities while reading a book. It can be seen, as is well known from eye movement studies, that the rate of visual moments as reflected by the rate of eye jumps, is relatively high, while rates of hearing, smelling, and proprioception are decreased. This fits the general idea that a reader is essentially a visual processor and that his attention in other sensory spheres is attenuated. However, rather than assuming that the attention to other spheres is attenuated by decreasing the amplitude of the signals from the other spheres or raising thresholds, it is instead assumed that the amount of attention in a particular sphere is mainly controlled by the frequency with which that particular sphere has input moments, i.e., by controlling the rate at which the sphere is monitored by the central processor.

Figure 8.3 shows the sensory organization while relaxing and listening to music. As can be seen, it is the auditory system which has a high rate of input moments and all other systems are relatively less active. If, instead of relaxed listening to music, intent listening for a footstep to fall was represented, the rate at which auditory moments occur might merely increase.

The general idea is clear enough so that Figs. 8.4 and 8.5 may now be considered. In each case the sensory modality most involved shows the highest rate of input moments. Likewise, the idea of compound sensory activities where several modalities are used extensively is evident in the example of watching television in Fig. 8.6, were both hearing and vision have high rates of processing as the watcher assimilates both the visual image and that which is heard over the sound channel.

Although the model is remarkably uncomplicated and explains many things simply, it also must not be forgotten that it is an information processing

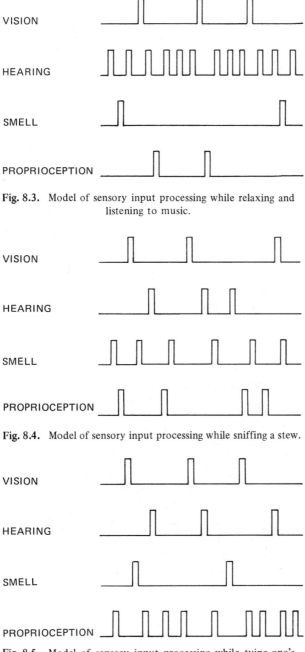

Fig. 8.3. Model of sensory input processing while relaxing and listening to music.

Fig. 8.4. Model of sensory input processing while sniffing a stew.

Fig. 8.5. Model of sensory input processing while tying one's shoes in the dark

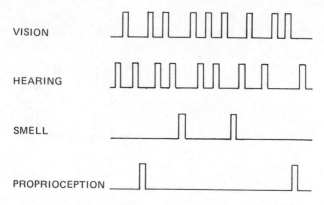

Fig. 8.6. Model of sensory input processing while watching television

model and, as such, understanding it lies not only in grasping its simplicity but also in grasping how it applies to informational consideration. One such consideration is the idea of alternative information processing strategies and the learning of particular patterns of information processing. Thus, engaging in a particular activity requires using a particularly well-learned pattern of input programming. For example, several particular television watchers might have identical rates of 4 eye jumps a second, 4 hearing input moments a second and only 1 smell moment and 1 proprioceptive moment. However, these might be combined in many different ways. One person might always follow a visual moment with an auditory moment, whereas another would always follow an auditory moment with a visual moment. A third person might have them randomly, resulting in no particular pattern. In each case, however, a particular sensory input structure would emerge and it would have its particular entropy value as a reflection of the degree of constraint in that structure. A further informational consideration, which carries us beyond present understanding, is that we must assume hierarchical units whose structural characteristic is that they are made of lower units from several sensory modalities. This means that earlier reference to a particular hierarchical level of vision which is made up of several visual information packages combined (Sec. 5.6), must be broadened to include a picture of informational units from several modalities combining to form broader sensory impressions. Thus, a sequence containing a particular smell, a particular sight, and a particular sound might make up a unit of information that makes one aware, for example, that dinner is ready. However, it is clear that the precise definition of such things is presently beyond understanding and that only the dim outline of the possibilities can be perceived now.

8.3. General Serial Model of Behavior

Thus far solely the sensory systems of the brain have been considered in constructing our model. By noticing that different rates of sensory processing have been allowed, the possibility of times when very little sensory information is being processed can be recognized. This means there would be many input moments in which there was no sensory input. In addition, cognitive, emotional, and memory functions to this point have been omitted. Each of these will be defined loosely and in a common sense way, ignoring that each must be further broken down and specified. This is not to deny the importance of more precise definitions, but rather to restrict the scope to going only as far as present knowledge admits.

In considering the contents of the stream of consciousness, as conceptualized by James (1950) and elaborated by Horn (1965) and Horowitz (1970), it is not difficult to conceive of psychological states that vary in the degree to which sensory, cognitive, emotional, and memory functions are combined. Thus, it is possible to conceive of a hunter, intently tracking his prey, as being totally absorbed in the sensory sphere and having virtually no cognitive nor memory function involved in his stream of consciousness. His stream of consciousness would not include much thinking, but would be almost purely sensory. Alternately, it is possible to conceive of an intensely cognitive activity, such as carrying out a chain of computations with simple numbers, in which the invividual would be so oblivious to his sensory world as to be unresponsive to many sensations. Finally, a very relaxed state of reverie might include almost only memories, with very little cognitive or sensory activity. Even though this classification of conscious activity is sketchy, it serves to make the point that input to the central processor is not only sensory; but that states of consciousness which draw heavily for their content on cognitive, emotional, or memory functions may also be considered. At this point it is not necessary to decide whether to think of these things as alternative "inputs" or to think of them as central activities that serially alternate with sensory inputs and with one another. Likewise, for the sake of simplicity, the place of motor activity will be ignored. Now, a

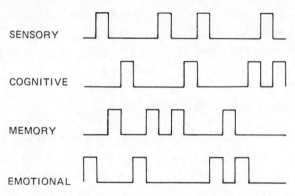

Fig. 8.7. General serial model of cortical processing.

complete model of serially processed behavior can be assembled; all the parts are there.

An assumption is to be made that only one of the four spheres (sensation, thought, emotion, and memory) may occupy the central processor at one moment; but that in the next moment any of the spheres may enter the central processor. The action of the processor is then one of moving a step at a time, and at each step of the way carrying out an action in one of these spheres. This can be best understood by reference to the same notation used to describe the sensory sphere above (Sec. 8.2). Figure 8.7 gives an example. Here, arbitrary assumptions must be made. Most of the time is assumed to be filled by one of the spheres; there is little time in which some of these all-encompassing activities are not being carried out. Since, the exact nature of the units is not certain, it is not known for certain whether a sensory unit is composed of several sensory moments, or whether thought must always be preceded by sensation. Considering a sensory evoked response, does the first wave represent the sensory input and the later waves the cognitive decision-making activity carried out upon the input, so that the evoked response wave is the tangible manifestation of a chain of behavior? (The wavelike nature of evoked responses and the many recent experiments associating different behavioral properties to the different parts of the evoked response wave are particularly intriguing here [Chapman, 1973].)

8.4 Implications of the Model

An examination of the structure of the behavior model shows that unique psychological moments, which can also be considered as momentary psychophysiological states, are being defined. According to Ashby (1963) *state* has a very widely applicable meaning, but is very precisely definable. The state of a mechanism is totally defined by knowing the immediately preceding state and the input at that moment. In considering the diagram of central processing in Fig. 8.7, each point along the horizontal (time) dimension can be thought of as defining a particular state, so that at any given moment it could be said, for example, "now we are in a cognitive moment which was just preceded by a moment of visual input" or "now we are in a moment of auditory input which was just preceded by a moment of memory." It is very important to notice that these moments are links of a chain and that the chain is behavior (that the structure of these units is what makes up behavior).

Just as in information hierarchies, there are higher levels to move to, here. When the levels of the individual units (just considered), which are psychological moments or which define unique momentary psychophysiological states, are linked into chains, the basis for unique *ongoing* psychophysiological "states" which are defined by the composition of the chain of momentary states, become apparent. The ongoing psychophysiological state is the relatively invariant chain of states over a longer period of time and is a higher unit of the information-bearing hierarchy. Thus, any particular ongoing psychophysiological state might be defined in terms of the composition of its links of momentary states. For example, in reading a book it might be found that there would be 3.2 sensory (almost all visual) moments, 2 cognitive moments and 1.6 memory moments per second. Again, just as there is a structure to the sensory sphere, so would there be a structure to the ongoing psychophysiological state, with it making a great deal difference in what order the units are arranged. These structured ongoing psychophysiological states would be unique to the particular activity in which the organism was engaged at a particular time. Thus, reading a book would result in a different structure from sitting in reverie or listening to a friend talk. The behavior model may be used to follow William James' ideas about the will (1950) with a definition of will as the capacity to program the structure of behavior to a particular end. Different states of consciousness (Fischer, 1971; Gaarder, 1971a; Tart, 1969), as achieved in so-called "altered" states of consciousness—the different levels of Yogi and Zen states, etc.—represent tangible differences in the programming of the person. This is an extension and specification of the work on the programming of behavior begun by Miller, Galanter, and Pribram (1960).

8.5. Recapitulation

A serial processing model of behavior has been described in which not only different sensory modalities, but also other different spheres of the mind must be processed serially by the brain. From this many psychological phenomena (such as the focusing of attention, the different states of mental organization associated with different behavioral activities, the nature of the exercise of will and the definition of states of consciousness), can be accounted for. Such investigation is justified by assuming it reaches in the right direction, even if it does not point directly to the mark.

9
SUMMARY

9.1. Introduction

The purpose of this chapter is to recapitulate the major points made in the book from the sharp focus of stating each as a simple fact or simple assumption. Whereas in the body of the book the method has been to build up to central ideas through providing proof, logic, and factual background, here the method is to state simply the major points in as clear a way as possible, to allow no misunderstanding about what is meant. There are twelve points to be made, with a certain amount of overlap which will be indicated. When a point is made, one or more of three reasons for accepting the point will be given. The first reason is because the point is in harmony with an apparently valid frame of reference, such as homeostatic frame of reference. The second reason for accepting a point is because of its demonstration through practical examples which force conclusions from already known facts. The third reason is from experimental facts which have been presented in the book. This recapitulation of the major points also serves as a summary of the book. At the beginning of the section stating each point, the place it is described in the book will be given in parentheses.

9.2. Point 1: Vision Is a Homeostatic Feedback System (Secs. 1.10–1.15)

Until recently, visual system models have tended to be organized as linear mechanistic models, with little attention being given to homeostatic feedback mechanisms. Now, however, the demonstrated ubiquity of homeostatic feedback mechanisms is increasingly being taken as presumptive evidence for their existence in any complex biosystem, such as the visual system. We may presume that homeostatic feedback mechanisms operate in the visual system from the perspective of the current apparently valid frame of reference of homeostatic feedback physiology. The visual system is homeostatically adaptive not only because vision regulates such processes as escaping danger and seeking nourishment, but also because visual regulation is essential to the adjustment of psychophysiological state—arousal level, specific excitations, etc.

However, this does not tell us where and how feedbacks operate within the system. One question is whether there are feedbacks between the eye and the brain, whether the brain can effect what the eye tells it. Because other major receptive organizations have been demonstrated to have connections between the central system and the peripheral receptor system we assume this possible in the eye. Also, it is possible to demonstrate such connections in trivial (from a holistic and perceptual standpoint) instances, such as pupil and lens homeostatic feedback mechanisms. The frame of reference of homeostatic feedback physiology suggests, however, that feedback has a crucial role in visual perception. The only currently practical way of studying this in humans is by studying eye movements. In one instance such a feedback in eye movements is self-evident: If one wishes to see something distinctly which is in his peripheral vision he turns his eye to bring the object to the greater acuity of the central retinal areas in and near the fovea. He has thereby used the feedback of eye movements to alter the retinal image and the input to the brain. The process is homeostatic because the internal equilibrium is maintained by being able to look where it is important to look. But once the eye has come to rest on the object of interest does vision cease to be mediated by a feedback?

Thus far we have established our first major point—that vision is a homeostatic feedback system—by reference to the current idea of the ubiquity of such systems and by reference to the obvious fedback in accessory visual functions such as pupil and lens adjustments.

We have also shown how eye movement can be a feedback, but we have not yet dealt with the instance of an eye fixating for a long time upon a viewed object. It is here that we move to our second major point, which will provide further evidence that vision is a homeostatic feedback system by showing that eye jumps represent a concrete means of providing a feedback.

9.3. Point 2: Eye Jumps Are a Feedback
(Secs. 1.16–1.22)

Even when the eye fixates an object, it continues to make small movements invisible to unaided inspection. These movements include abrupt jumps that occur several times a second. Since these jumps change visual input by abruptly changing the retinal image, they could be a feedback. If these small jumps represent a feedback from the brain to the eye which functions to partly control the input to the eye, then it would be expected when the visual stimulus viewed by the eye is changed, that the eye jumps would also be changed. This would be a feedback because visual input was differentially changed by the brain output of eye movement altering the retinal image. On the other hand, if eye jumps had no feedback function, they might be expected to show no relation to the visual stimulus. Experiments show unequivocally that eye jumps are different with different stimuli and therefore eye jumps can be a feedback. Point 3 and 6 (Secs. 9.4 & 9.7) will show *how* the eye jump is a feedback by demonstrating specific consequences of specific eye jumps. In other words, by showing how different eye jumps produce different input, it will be shown that eye jumps do function as a feedback.

9.4. Point 3: Eye Jumps Are Step Functions
Giving Evoked Cortical Responses
(Secs. 2.4–2.6)

Each jump of the eye causes an abrupt displacement of the retinal image on the eye. This abrupt change is termed a "step function" in engineering and would be expected to produce a chain of transient responses in any receptive system. In fact, there is an evoked response elicited in the visual area of the cortex by eye jumps. This evoked response is produced only by the change of the eye jumping, without any objective change of the stimulus, but is nonetheless very similar to evoked responses elicited by the change of flashing light stimuli. In other words, in spite of the fact that the outside stimulus itself remains constant, the brain-controlled jump of the eye, by shifting the retinal image of the stimulus, causes a transient response in the form of a typical cortical evoked response.

9.5. Point 4: Eye Jumps Are Related to the Internal Pacing Mechanisms of the Brain (Secs. 3.3, 3.5, & 3.6)

Because the brain orders the eye to jump, the brain thereby causes itself to be stimulated by the resultant retinal image change and it is, therefore, partly controlling its own input. There are also other ways in which the brain controls its own input, in other sensory modalities by using self-pacing mechanisms of intermittency. These mechanisms can most vividly be pictured by saying there are brief moments when the brain will take in a given stimulus sandwiched between other moments in which the brain's central processor is unreceptive to the stimulus but when the stimulus may be stored to wait another input moment. The cyclical alpha rhythm of the brain is closely related to these input pacing mechanisms. It is, therefore, important that eye jumps, which partly regulate visual input, are shown experimentally to be closely related to the phase of the alpha rhythm wave cycle. Through the linkage of alpha rhythm, we have a relation between eye jumps as a pacer of visual input and other sensory input pacing mechanisms. Technically, it is of great importance that the jump of the eye is the only sharp and discrete external manifestation of the internal event of input moments now available.

9.6. Point 5: Beta Rhythm Has Exactly Twice the Frequency of Alpha Rhythm (Sec. 3.4)

The form of the model evolving here leads to the prediction that beta brain waves (20Hz) should have exactly twice the frequency of alpha brain waves (10Hz). One reason for this is that the temporal dimensionality of units (Sec. 9.10, Point 9) allows for temporally larger units to be constructed of several temporally smaller units. This also predicts larger and smaller units at either end of this continuum—for 5Hz theta waves which are exactly half of alpha frequency and for 40Hz "low voltage fast activity" which is exactly twice beta frequency, since still larger compound units and still smaller basic units are anticipated.

9.7. Point 6: Eye Jump Effects Can Be Concretely Visualized (Secs. 4.5-4.9)

From the inescapable simple knowledge of what happens when the eye jumps, it is possible to construct pictorial representations simulating exactly the effect of eye jumps on the retinal image (Figs. 4.3, 4.4, 4.6, & 4.7). When the edge of an object is imaged on the retina there are five definable conditions present after a small eye jump takes place:

1. There is a retinal area to one side of the edge in which no change takes place.
2. There is a sharp boundary where the edge was imaged *before* the jump took place.
3. There is a band of change in which the area to one side of the edge was present before the eye jump and the area to the other side of the edge is present after the jump.
4. There is a sharp boundary where the edge is imaged *after* the jump takes place.
5. There is another retinal area on the opposite side from Condition 1 where no change has taken place.

Simple geometric analysis shows that the sets of changed edges generated by eye jump vectors in particular directions are unique to the eye jump vector. This supplements the proof of homeostatic feedback (Secs. 9.2 & 9.3) since it can be seen that there is a unique effect of the brain-controlled eye jump feedback which controls the nature of the brain's input. In other words, we are assuming at a particular moment a particular visual scene, with its image focused on the retina and with the visual information in the scene already partly assimilated by the brain. We are then asserting that the way in which the visual information will continue to be assimilated will be controlled by the brain through the feedback of eye jumps, which determines the particular type of edge template to be presented to the central system through the determination of the eye jump vector.

The same effects instantaneously produced by eye jumps are also more continuously produced by the drift of the eye during fixation. This may also contribute to the contents of a given eye jump package and is also controlled by feedback of eye movement, but the abrupt change defining the package's temporal boundaries comes from eye jumps as shown in the next section.

9.8. Point 7: Eye Jumps Cause the
      Packaging of Visual Information
      (Secs. 5.6, 6.2, & 6.3)

The points made to here have shown that vision is a homeostatic process in which eye jumps function as a feedback. This feedback is not continuous, however, since eye jumps are abrupt, discontinuous step functions and the resultant evoked response is a transient phenomenon. The unique sets of edge information considered in the last point (Sec. 9.7) are the result of the eye jumps. The sets of edge information exist on the retinal image and are what is transmitted to the visual cortex in the evoked responses linked to the eye jumps. The information coded in the electrical activity of the evoked response is a "package" of information because it has boundaries—temporal and spatial—within the nervous system. This conclusion is partly justified by the cybernetic frame of reference in which categories of continuous versus discontinuous are distinguished.

9.9. Point 8: Bioinformation Must Be Hierarchically Organized (Secs. 5.3, 5.5, & 5.6)

Two alternative schemes of information organization can be contrasted. In the nonhierarchical form, represented by a photographic plate, with discrete grains of silver compounds, the nature of the organization of light and dark is entirely imposed arbitrarily from without by the organization of the external image to be represented. In contrast, hierarchical forms of information represented by a printed language, are constrained by an elaborate system of rules in which alphabetic letters are built into words, which are built into sentences, and so forth. Without this elaborate hierarchical organization, a language cannot carry information.

Since it is only recently that the concept of hierarchical information organization has been widely appreciated, it has often been implicitly assumed until now that bioinformation was organized nonhierarchically. When the alternatives are weighed, however, it seems likely that bio-information, as conveyed by living nervous systems, would be hierarchically organized, with increasing size of hierarchical units being accomplished through increasing the temporal duration occupied by a unit, so that time becomes the dimension in which hierarchical unit size is expressed. The visual system is a particularly good example from which to consider the question of bioinformation organization which will be done in the next point, showing why eye jump packages are part of the hierarchy.

9.10. Point 9: Eye Jump Packages of Visual Information Are Units in the Hierarchy of Visual Information (Secs. 5.6 & 6.3)

Since visual information is divided into packages by the discrete discontinuous step function jumps of the eye, and since visual information is assumed to be organized in hierarchical structure of discontinuous units in a way analogous to language, it is most parsimonious and logical in this situation to assume that eye jump packages of visual information are intermediate units in the hierarchy of visual information processing. Just as the alphabetic letter is the lowest unit of language, so may a nerve spike discharge be assumed the lowest unit of bioinformation.

In viewing a scene with gross eye jumps it may be assumed that the emergent reconstruction of the scene as a percept is a higher order unit of the hierarchy analogous to a sentence. For instance, the package of visual information taken in with each fixation of the eye would be an intermediate order unit of the hierarchy (such as a word); the nerve spikes patterned into the eye jump package would be analogous to the lowest order unit of letters making up the word.

9.11. Point 10: Bioinformation Organization Has Effects across Sensory Modalities (Secs. 7.2, 7.4, & 7.5)

This means there are structural information processing relationships across modalities. Once it is assumed that bioinformation is organized in discontinuous temporally discrete units, it becomes apparent that there must be definable relations between these units from different sense modalities. For example, when the visual information packages associated with eye jumps are processed by the cortex, it is possible by experiment to tell what relation auditory signal processing bears to this. Elementary evaluation of the set of possibilities in basic programming shows that auditory processing could either be serial (in sequence with visual processing), parallel (simultaneous with visual processing), or independent (unrelated to visual processing).

A further crucial point, however, is that not only do we expect experimental relations between auditory and visual processing signals, but in addition we assume the information carried in these signals must have a hierarchical organizational structure which can be defined. The importance of this is in prescribing an organizing principle for neurophysiological experiments around the concept of hierarchical information with structured intermodality relations.

9.12. Point 11: Sensory Input from Different Modalities Is Probably Serially Processed (Sec. 7.5)

Experiments point tentatively toward the relation between auditory and visual information processing being serial in nature, so that if the central processing system is processing fresh visual data, it cannot simultaneously be processing fresh auditory data, and vice versa.

9.13. Point 12: A Serial Processing Model of Behavior Is a Likely One of a Limited Number of Possibilities (Secs. 8.2 & 8.3)

From consideration of the points made previously, it is obvious that a model that accounts for behavior must account for the organization of information required to achieve that behavior. In particular, the sensory input systems must either be organized to continually present information to central processing or to do so discontinuously. Evidence favors this being discontinuous. A discontinuous processing system immediately implies rules governing intermodality processing, and evidence favors serial processing. A serial processing model of behavior is one in which only one sense modality may be centrally processed at a time. By assuming different rates of central processing, the model accounts for differing information processing capacities associated with different levels of arousal. By assuming differential relative rates of information processing between sensory modalities, the model accounts for the focusing of attention. By including cognitive, mnemonic, and affective processing as alternatives to sensory processing, the model accounts for other mental spheres as well.

By acknowledging the hierarchical structure of bioinformation, the model allows for higher informational units which are composed of subunits from several modalities, such as hearing and vision, for example, or which have components from both affective and cognitive spheres, for another example.

When chains of these units are conceived as programs, one has a frame of reference to account for different states of consciousness as made of different processing programs with particular chains of processing units for the particular program.

BIBLIOGRAPHY

Alpern, M. Eye movements. In D. Jameson and L. M. Hurvich (Eds.), *Handbook of sensory physiology*. Vol. VII/4. *Visual psychophysics*. Berlin: Springer-Verlag, 1972.

Arbib, M. A. *Brains, machines, and mathematics*. New York: McGraw-Hill Book Company, 1964.

Armington, J. C., Gaarder, K., & Schick, A. Variation of spontaneous ocular and occipital responses with stimulus patterns. *Journal of the Optical Society of America, 57,* 1967, 1534–1538.

Ashby, W. R. *Design for a brain: The origin of adaptive behaviour*. New York: John Wiley & Sons, Inc., 1960.

Ashby, W. R. *An introduction to cybernetics*. New York: John Wiley & Sons, Inc., 1963.

Averbach, E., & Sperling, G. Short term storage of information in vision. In C. Cherry (Ed.), *Information theory. Fourth London Symposium*. London: Butterworth & Co., 1961.

Barlow, J. S. Evoked responses in relation to visual perception and oculomotor reaction times in man. *Annals of the New York Academy of Sciences, 112,* 1964, 432–467.

Beeler, G. W., Jr. *Stochastic processes in the human eye movement control system*. (Doctoral thesis, California Institute of Technology) Ann Arbor, Michigan: University Microfilms, 1965, Film # 65-11, 065.

Bertelson, P. Central intermittency twenty years later. *Quarterly Journal of Experimental Psychology, 18,* 1966, 153–163.

Bickford, R. G., Jacobson, J. L., & Cody, D. T. R. Nature of average evoked potentials to sound and other stimuli in man. *Annals of the New York Academy of Sciences, 112,* 1964, 204–223.

Bickford, R. G., & Klass, D. W. Eye movement and the electroencephalogram. In M. B. Bender (Ed.), *The oculomotor system*. New York: Harper and Row Publishers, Inc., 1964.

143

Biersdorf, W. R., & Nakamura, Z. Electroencephalogram potentials evoked by hemi-retinal stimulation. *Experientia, 27,* 1971, 402–403.

Birdwhistell, R. L. *Kinesics and context: Essays on body motion communication.* New York: Ballantine Books, Inc., 1970.

Boernstein, W. S. Optic perception and optic imageries in man. Their roots and relations studied from the viewpoint of biology. *International Journal of Neurology, 6,* 1967, 147–181.

Boynton, R. M. Retinal contrast mechanisms. In F. A. Young & D. B. Lindsley (Eds.), *Early experience and visual information processing in perceptual and reading disorders.* Washington, D.C.: National Academy of Sciences, 1970.

Brown, B. Recognition of aspects of consciousness through association with EEG alpha activity represented by a light signal. *Psychophysiology, 6,* 1970, 442–452.

Callaway, E., III, & Yeager, C. L. Relationship between reaction time and electroencephalographic alpha phase. *Science, 132,* 1960, 1765–1766.

Cantril, H. *The why of man's experience.* New York: Macmillan Company, 1950.

Chapman, R. M. Evoked potentials of the brain related to thinking. In F. J. McGuigan & R. A. Schoonover (Eds.), *The psychophysiology of thinking.* New York: Academic Press Inc., 1973.

Chase, R. A. An information-flow model of the organization of motor activity. Part I. Transduction, transmission and central control of sensory information. Part II. Sampling, central processing, and utilization of sensory information. *Journal of Nervous and Mental Disease, 140,* 1965, 239–251; 334–350.

Clark, J. H. Adaptive machines in psychiatry. In N. Wiener & J. P. Schade (Eds.), *Nerve, brain and memory models.* Amsterdam: Elsevier Publishing Company, 1963.

Cohn, R. Differential cerebral processing of noise and verbal stimuli. *Science, 172,* 1971, 599–601.

Conant, R. C. The information transfer required in regulatory processes. *IEEE Transactions on Systems Science and Cybernetics,* SSC-5, 1969, 334–338.

Creutzfeldt, O. D., Watanabe, S., & Lux, H. D. Relations between EEG phenomena and potentials of single cortical cells. II. Spontaneous and convulsoid activity. *Electroencephalography and Clinical Neurophysiology, 20,* 1966, 19–37.

Cunitz, R. J., & Steinman, R. M. Comparison of saccadic eye movements during fixation and reading. *Vision Research, 9,* 1969, 683–693.

Davson, H. (Ed.) *The Eye.* New York: Academic Press Inc., 1970.

de Valois, R. L. Neural processing of visual information. In R. W. Russel (Ed.), *Frontiers in physiological psychology.* New York: Academic Press Inc., 1966.

Dewey, J. *Human nature and conduct.* New York: Henry Holt and Company, Inc., 1922.

Ditchburn, R. W., & Ginsborg, B. L. Involuntary eye movements during fixation. *Journal of Physiology, 119,* 1953, 1–17.

Farley, B. G., & Clark, W. A. Activity in networks of neuron-like elements. In C. Cherry (Ed.), *Information theory. Fourth London Symposium.* London: Butterworth & Co., 1961.

Fender, D. H. Control mechanisms of the eye. *Scientific American,* July 1964, 2–11.

Festinger, L. Eye movements and perception. In P. Bach-y-Rita & C. C. Collins (Eds.), *The control of eye movements.* New York: Academic Press Inc., 1971.

Festinger, L., Burnham, C. A., Ono, H., & Bamber, D. Efference and the conscious experience of perception. *Journal of Experimental Psychology,* **74**, 1967, 1-36.

Fischer, R. A cartography of the ecstatic and meditative states. *Science,* **174**, 1971, 897-904.

Flavell, J. H., & Draguns, J. A. Microgenetic approach to perception and thought. *Psychological Bulletin,* **54**, 1957, 197-234.

Fox, S. S., & O'Brien, J. H. Duplication of evoked potential waveform by curve of probability of firing of a single cell. *Science,* **147**, 1965, 888-890.

Gaarder, K. Relating a component of physiological nystagmus to visual display. *Science,* **132**, 1960, 471-472.

Gaarder, K. Alternative physiological mechanisms of information transfer between the retina and the brain in visual perception. *British Journal of Physiological Optics,* **20**, 1963, 1-7.

Gaarder, K. A conceptual model of sleep. *Archives of General Psychiatry,* **14**, 1966, 253-260 (a).

Gaarder, K. Fine eye movements during inattention. *Nature,* **209**, 1966, 83 (b).

Gaarder, K. Transmission of edge information in the human visual system. *Nature,* **212**, 1966, 321-323 (c).

Gaarder, K. Mechanisms in fixation saccadic eye movements. *British Journal of Physiological Optics,* **24**, 1967, 28-44 (a).

Gaarder, K. Some patterns of fixation saccadic eye movements. *Psychonomic Science,* **7**, 1967, 145-146 (b).

Gaarder, K. Interpretive study of evoked responses elicited by gross saccadic eye movements. *Perceptual and Motor Skills,* **27**, 1968, 683-703 (Monograph supplement 2-V27).

Gaarder, K. A theoretical and experimental examination of audiovisual interaction. *Perceptual and Motor Skills,* **29**, 1969, 23-33.

Gaarder, K. Eye movements and perception. In F. A. Young & D. B. Lindsley (Eds.), *Early experience and visual information processing in perceptual and reading disorders.* Washington, D.C.: National Academy of Sciences, 1970.

Gaarder, K. Control of states of consciousness. I. Attainment through control of psychophysiological variables. *Archives of General Psychiatry,* **25**, 1971, 429-435 (a).

Gaarder, K. Control of states of consciousness. II. Attainment through external feedback augmenting control of psychophysiological variables. *Archives of General Psychiatry,* **25**, 1971, 436-441 (b).

Gaarder, K., Alterman, A., & Kropfl, W. The relation of the phase-locked saccade-linked component of alpha rhythm to change of stimulus illuminances. *Psychonomic Science,* **5**, 1966, 445-446 (a).

Gaarder, K., Koresko, R., & Kropfl, W. The phasic relation of a component of alpha rhythm to fixation saccadic eye movements. *Electronencephalography and Clinical Neurophysiology,* **21**, 1966, 544-551 (b).

Gaarder, K., Krauskopf, J., Graf, V., Kropfl, W., & Armington, J. C. Averaged brain activity following saccadic eye movements. *Science,* **146**, 1964, 1481-1483.

Gaarder, K., Silverman, J., Pfefferbaum, D., Pfefferbaum, L., & King, C. Infra-red method for assessment of small and large eye movements in clinical experiments. *Perceptual and Motor Skills,* **25**, 1967, 473-484.

Gaarder. K., & Speck, L. The quasi-harmonic relations of alpha and beta peaks in the power spectrum. *Brain Research,* **4**, 1967, 110–112.

Galambos, R., Sheatz, G., & Vernier, V. G. Electrophysiological correlates of a conditioned response in cats. *Science,* **123**, 1956, 376–377.

Gibson, J. J. The senses considered as perceptual systems. *Science,* **155**, 1966, 1232–1233.

Graham, C. H. (Ed.) *Vision and visual perception.* New York: John Wiley & Sons, Inc., 1965.

Granit, R. *The basis of motor control.* New York: Academic Press Inc., 1970.

Harmon, L. D., & Lewis, E. R. Neural modeling. *Physiological Reviews,* **46**, 1966, 513–591.

Harter, M. R. Excitability cycles and cortical scanning: A review of two hypotheses of central intermittency in perception. *Psychological Bulletin,* **68**, 1967, 47–58.

Harter, M. R., Seiple, W. H., & Salmon, L. Binocular summation of visually evoked responses to pattern stimuli in humans. *Vision Research,* **13**, 1973, 1433–1446.

Hebb, D. O. *The organization of behavior.* New York: John Wiley & Sons, Inc., 1949.

Hebbard, F. W., & Fischer, R. Effect of psilocybin, LSD, and mescaline on small, involuntary eye movements. *Psychopharmacologia,* **9**, 1966, 146–156.

Held, R. Exposure history as a factor in maintaining stability of perception and coordination. *Journal of Nervous and Mental Disease,* **132**, 1961, 26–32.

Hernandez-Peon, R., Scherrer, H., & Jouvet, M. Modification of electrical activity in cochlear nucleus during "attention" in unanesthetized cats. *Science,* **123**, 1956, 331–332.

Hirsch, I. Auditory perception of temporal order. *Journal of the Acoustical Society of America,* **31**, 1959, 759–767.

Hochberg, J. E. *Perception.* Englewood Cliffs, N. J.: Prentice-Hall, Inc., 1964.

Horn, G. Physiological and psychological aspects of selective perception. *Advances in Animal Behavior,* **1**, 1965, 155–215.

Horowitz, M. J. *Image formation and cognition.* New York: Appleton-Century-Crofts, Inc., 1970.

Hubel, D. N., & Wiesel, T. N. Receptive fields and functional architecture in two non-striate visual areas of the cat. *Journal of Neurophysiology,* **28**, 1965, 228–289.

Iberall, A., & McCulloch, W. S. 1967 Behavioral model of man. His chains revealed. *Currents in Modern Biology,* **1/5**, 1968, 337–352.

James, W. *Principles of psychology.* New York: Dover Publication, Inc., 1950

Jameson, D., & Hurvich, L. M. (Eds.), *Handbook of sensory physiology.* Vol. VII/4. *Visual psychophysics.* Berlin: Springer-Verlag, 1972.

John, E. R. Switchboard versus statistical theories of learning and memory. *Science,* **177**, 1972, 850–864.

John, E. R., Herrington, R. N., & Sutton, S. Information delivery and the sensory evoked potential. *Science,* **155**, 1967, 1436–1442.

Jones, R. W. *Principles of biological regulation: An introduction to feedback systems.* New York: Academic Press Inc., 1973.

Kamiya, J. Operant control of the EEG alpha rhythm and some of its reported effects on consciousness. In C. T. Tart (Ed.), *Altered states of consciousness.* New York: John Wiley & Sons, Inc., 1969.

Kasamatsu, A., & Hirai, T. An electroencephalographic study on the zen meditation (zazen). *Folia Psychiatrica and Neurologica Japonica,* 20, 1966, 315-336.

Krauskopf, J., Graf, V., & Gaarder, K. Lack of inhibition during involuntary saccades. *American Journal of Psychology,* 79, 1966, 73-81.

Kristofferson, A. B. Attention and psychophysical time. *Acta Psychologica,* 27, 1967, 93-100.

Langley, L. L. *Homeostasis.* New York: Reinhold Publishing Corporation, 1965.

Lewin, K. *Principles of topological psychology.* New York: McGraw Hill Book Company, 1936.

Lindsley, D. B. Psychological phenomena and the electroencephalogram. *Electroencephalography and Clinical Neurophysiology,* 4, 1952, 443-456.

Lipshutz, S. *Theory and problems of set theory and related topics.* New York: Schaum Outline Series, Schaum Publishing, 1964.

Luborsky, L., Rick, R., Phoenix, D., & Fisher, C. Eye fixation behavior as a function of awareness. *Journal of Personality,* 36, 1968, 1-20.

Luriia, A. R., Pravdina-Vinarskaia, E. N., & Yarbus, A. L. Eye movement mechanisms in normal and pathological vision. *Voprosy Psikhologii,* 1961, No. 5. (Abstracted in: *Soviet Psychology and Psychiatry,* 2, 1964, 28-39.)

Mackworth, N. H. A stand camera for line of sight recording. *Perception and Psychophysiology,* 2, 1967, 119-127.

Mackworth, N. H., & Bruner, J. S. *Selecting visual information during recognition by children and adults.* Unpublished monograph, Harvard University Center for Cognitive Studies, July 1966.

Marshall, W. H., & Talbot, S. A. Recent evidence for neural mechanisms in vision leading to a general theory of sensory acuity. In H. Kluver (Ed.), *Biological symposia. Vol. III. Visual mechanisms.* Lancaster, Penn.: Jaques Cattell Press, Inc., 1942.

Matin, L. Eye movements and perceived visual direction. In D. Jameson and L. M. Hurvich (Eds.), *Handbook of sensory physiology.* Vol. VII/4. *Visual psychophysics.* Berlin: Springer-Verlag, 1972.

Maynard, D. M. Simpler networks. *Annals of the New York Academy of Sciences,* 193, 1972, 59-72.

Mayr, O. *The origins of feedback control.* Cambridge, Mass.: M.I.T. Press, 1970.

Mayzner, M. S., Tresselt, M. E., & Helfer, M. S. A provisional model of visual information processing with sequential inputs. *Psychonomic Monograph Supplements,* 2, 1967, 91-108.

Mead, G. H. *The philosophy of the act.* Chicago: University of Chicago Press, 1938.

Miller, G. A., Galanter, E., & Pribram, K. H. *Plans and the structure of behavior.* New York: Holt, Rinehart and Winston, Inc., 1960.

Millodot, M. Foveal and extra-foveal acuity with and without stabilized retinal images. *British Journal of Physiological Optics,* 23, 1966, 75-106.

Minsky, M., and Papert, S. *Perceptrons.* Cambridge, Mass.: M.I.T. Press, 1969.

Moore, G. P., Perkel, D. H., & Segundo, J. P. Statistical analysis and functional interpretation of neuronal spike data. *Annual Review of Physiology,* 28, 1966, 493-522.

Mulholland, T., & Evans, C. R. Oculomotor function and the alpha activation cycle. *Nature,* 211, 1966, 1278-1279.

Murphy, G. *Personality: A biosocial approach to origins and structure.* New York: Basic Books, Inc., Publishers, 1966.

Navweps OP3000. *Weapons systems fundamentals: Synthesis of systems.* Vol. 3. Washington, D.C.: United States Government Printing Office, 1963.

Noton, D., & Stark, L. Eye movements and visual perception. *Scientific American,* **224,** 1971, 34–43 (a).

Noton, D., & Stark, L. Scanpaths in eye movements during pattern perception. *Science,* **171,** 1971, 308–311 (b).

Palmer, R. D., Visual acuity and excitement. *Psychosomatic Medicine,* **28,** 1966, 364–374.

Palmer, R. D. Visual acuity and stimulus-seeking behavior. *Psychosomatic Medicine,* **32,** 1970, 277–284.

Pattee, H. H. (Ed.) *Hierarchy theory: The challenge of complex systems.* New York: George Braziller, Inc., 1973.

Picton, T. W., Hillyard, S. A., Galambos, R., & Schiff, M. Human auditory attention: A central or peripheral process? *Science,* **173,** 1971, 351–353.

Poggio, G. F., & Viernstein, L. J. Time series analysis of impulse sequences of thalamic somatic sensory neurons. *Journal of Neurophysiology,* **27,** 1964, 517–545.

Polanyi, M. Life's irreducible structure. *Science,* **160,** 1968, 1308–1312.

Pollen, D. A., Lee, J. R., & Taylor, J. H. How does the striate cortex begin the reconstruction of the visual world? *Science,* **173,** 1971, 74–77.

Polyak, S. L. *The retina.* Chicago: University of Chicago Press, 1941.

Powers, W. T. Feedback: Beyond behaviorism. *Science,* **179,** 1973, 351–356.

Powers, W. T., Clark, R. K., & McFarland, R. L. A general feedback theory of human behavior. Parts I and II. *Perceptual and Motor Skills,* 1960, **7,** 71–88; 309–323, (Monograph supplements 1-VII and 3-VII).

Ratliff, F. *Mach bands.* San Francisco: Holden Day, 1965.

Reiner, J. M. *The organism as an adaptive control system.* Englewood Cliffs, N.J.: Prentice-Hall, Inc., 1968.

Remond, A., Lesevre, N., & Torres, F. Étude chronotopographique de l'activité occipitale moyenne recueillie sur le scalp chez l'homme en relation avec les deplacements du regard (complexe lambda). *Revue Neurologique,* **113,** 1965, 193–226.

Rhodes, J. M., Lanoir, J., Saier, J., & Naquet, R. Etude des reponses evoquees par les mouvements des yeux le long de la voie visuelle. *Revue Neurologique,* **107,** 1962, 178–187.

Riggs, L. A., Armington, J. C., & Ratliff, F. Motions of the retinal image during fixation. *Journal of the Optical Society of America,* **44,** 1954, 315–321.

Ritow, I. *A servomechanism primer.* Garden City, N. Y.: Dolphin Books, Doubleday & Company, Inc., 1963.

Ruchkin, D. S., & John, E. R. Evoked potential correlates of generalization. *Science,* **153,** 1966, 209–211.

Ruesch, J., & Bateson, G. *Communication: The social matrix of psychiatry.* New York: W. W. Norton & Company, Inc., 1951.

Schilder, P. *The image and appearance of the human body.* New York: International Universities Press, Inc., 1950.

Schmidt, M., & Kristofferson, A. B. Discrimination of successiveness: A test of a model of attention. *Science,* **139,** 1963, 112–113.

Scott, D. F., & Bickford, R. G. Electrophysiologic studies during scanning and passive eye movements in humans. *Science,* 155, 1967, 101-102.

Scott, P., & Williams, K. G. A note on temporal coding as a mechanism in sensory perception. *Information and Control,* 2, 1959, 380-383.

Shannon, C. E. *The mathematical theory of communication.* Urbana, Illinois: University of Illinois Press, 1963. (Originally published: *Bell System Technical Journal,* 1948, 27, 379-423; 623-656.)

Silverman, J., & Gaarder, K. Rates of saccadic eye movement and size judgements of normal and schizophrenics. *Perceptual and Motor Skills,* 25, 1967, 661-667.

Singer, J. L., Greenberg, S., & Antrobus, J. S. Looking with the mind's eye: Experimental studies of ocular motility during daydreaming and mental arithmetic. *Transactions of the New York Academy of Sciences, Series II,* 33, 1971, 694-709.

Skavenski, A. A. Inflow as a source of extraretinal eye portion. *Vision Research,* 12, 1972, 221-229.

Sokolov, Y. N. *Perception and the conditioned reflex.* (Translated by S. Waydenfeld) New York: Macmillan Company, 1963.

Solley, C. M., & Murphy, G. *Development of the perceptual world.* New York: Basic Books, Inc., Publishers, 1960.

Stark, L. *Neurological control systems.* New York: Plenum Press, 1968.

Steinman, R. M. Effect of target size, luminance, and color on monocular fixation. *Journal of the Optical Society of America,* 55, 1965, 1158-1165.

Steinman, R. M., Cunitz, R. J., & Timberlake, G. T. Voluntary control of microsaccades during maintained monocular fixation. *Science,* 155, 1967, 1577-1579.

Steinman, R. M., Haddad, G. M., Skavenski, A. A., & Wyman, D. Miniature eye movement. *Science,* 181, 1973, 810-819.

Sutton, S., Tueting, P., Zubin, J., & John, E. R. Information delivery and the sensory evoked potential. *Science,* 155, 1967, 1436-1439.

Tart, C. T. (Ed.) *Altered states of consciousness.* New York: John Wiley & Sons, Inc. 1969.

Thomas, E. L. Movements of the eye. *Scientific American,* 219, 1968, 88-95.

Thomas, H. B. G. On the feedback regulation of choice behavior. *International Journal of Man-Machine Studies,* 2, 1970, 235-266.

Tinker, M. A. Recent studies of eye movements in reading. *Psychological Bulletin,* 55, 1958, 300-307.

Uttal, W. R. Do compound evoked potentials reflect psychological codes? *Psychological Bulletin,* 64, 1965, 377-392.

von Bertalanffy, L. *Robots, men and minds.* New York: George Braziller, Inc., 1967.

von Bertalanffy, L. *General systems theory.* New York: George Braziller, Inc., 1968.

von Foerster, H. The responsibility of competence. In *Cybernetic techniques in brain research and the educational process.* Washington, D. C.: American Society for Cybernetics, 1971.

von Holst, E. Relations between the central nervous system and the peripheral organs. *British Journal of Animal Behaviour,* 2, 1954, 89-94.

Weber, R. B., & Daroff, R. B. Corrective movements following refixation saccades: Type and control system analysis. *Vision Research,* 12, 1972, 467-476.

Wells, H., & Schmaustwein, H. How can you be so naive? *Artorga,* Communications 112-113, 1968, 1-18.

Wender, P. H. Vicious and virtuous circles: The role of deviation amplifying feedback in the origin and perpetuation of behavior. *Psychiatry, 31,* 1968, 309-324.

Werblin, F. S. Functional organization of the vertebrate retina: Sharpening up in space intensity. *Annals of the New York Academy of Sciences, 193,* 1972, 72-85.

Westwater, F. L. *Electronic computers.* London: English Universities Press, 1962.

White, C. T. Temporal numerosity and the psychological unit of duration. *Psychological Monographs, 77,* 1963, 1-37.

Whyte, L. L., Wilson, A. G., & Wilson, D. (Eds.) *Hierarchical structures.* New York: American Elsevier Publishing Company, 1969.

Wiener, N. *Cybernetics or control and communication in the animal and the machine.* Cambridge, Mass.: M.I.T. Press, 1948.

Worden, F. G. Attention and auditory electrophysiology. *Progress in Physiological Psychology, 1,* 1966, 46-116.

Yarbus, A. L. *Eye movements and vision.* (Translated by B. Haigh) New York: Plenum Press, 1967.

Young, L. R. Measuring eye movements. *American Journal of Medical Electronics, 2,* 1963, 300-307.

Young, L. R., & Stark, L. Variable feedback experiments using a sampled data model for eye tracking movements. *IEEE Transactions on Human Factors in Electronics,* HFE-4, 1963, 38-51.

Zuber, B. L., & Stark, L. Saccadic suppression: Elevation of visual threshold associated with saccadic eye movements. *Experimental Neurology, 16,* 1966, 65-79.

Zuber, B. L., Stark, L., & Cook, G. Microsaccades and the velocity-amplitude relationship for saccadic eye movements. *Science, 150,* 1965, 1459-1460.

NAME INDEX

Numbers in italics refer to the pages on which the complete references are cited.

SUBJECT INDEX

Adaptation, 1-3, 12-15, 31, 95, 136
Alpha brain waves, 47-51, 55-57, 98-99, 138
Analogy
    to auditory system, 18-19
    to computer information processing, 59-63, 79
    of eye jumps and stimulus onset, 38, 43-44
    of Koch's postulates, 11, 19-20
    to language, 76, 80-86, 88, 91-94, 104, 140, 141
    of ocean and brain waves, 35-37
    of photographs and percepts, 16-18, 64-76, 89, 96, 138
    in reasoning, 9-10
    of stimulus orientation to eye movement changes, 29, 30
    to television scanning, 105
Arousal, physiological, 13, 50, 136, 142
Attention, 101, 126-128, 134, 142
Audiovisual interaction, 99, 107-108, 115-134, 141
Auditory system, 20, 21, 107-108, 113-134
Averaging (*see* Computer of averaged transients)

Beta brain waves, 46, 51, 52, 138
Biofeedback (*see* Feedback, external psychophysiological)

Central intermittency (*see* Cortical excitability cycles)
Chains, 23, 45, 52, 74-76, 81, 83, 84, 87-89, 91-94, 96, 98, 105, 115, 131, 133, 142
Computer of averaged transients (CAT), 33-39, 56

Constraint, 83-85, 100, 130, 140
Continuous information processing, 17, 33, 43, 46, 47, 59-63, 111-112, 139, 140
Cortical excitability cycles, 44, 138
Cybernetics, 2-3, 102, 126, 140
Cycles, 49, 50, 54, 57, 96, 98, 104, 105, 138

Discontinuous information processing, 33, 37, 39, 43-51, 56, 57, 59-63, 71, 72, 76, 82, 84, 87-89, 92, 94, 96, 97, 99, 108-115, 123, 125, 139-141
Discrimination of successiveness, 113

Entropy, 100, 101, 130
Evoked response, 33-37, 39-44, 55-56, 96-99, 103, 104, 109, 113, 114, 132, 137, 139, 140
Eye movements
    changing retinal image, 1, 20, 21, 23, 24, 28-31, 41, 43, 63-76, 95-96, 99, 104, 109, 112, 136-140
    criticisms of eye jump model, 42-43, 101-106
    as feedback (*see* Feedback of eye movements)
    fixation drift type, 25, 70, 95-96, 99, 103-105, 113, 139
    fixation type, 14, 15, 22, 24-26, 28, 29, 39, 41, 48, 64-70, 91-104, 112-123, 136-138
    jumps and alpha, 51, 55, 56, 101
    jump elicited electroretinograms, 41
    jumps evoking responses, 39-44, 55-56, 96-98, 103, 104, 109, 113, 114, 132, 137, 139, 140